Mechanical Ventilation
MANUAL

EDITED BY:

SUHAIL RAOOF, MD, FACP, FCCP

ASSISTANT PROFESSOR OF MEDICINE
STATE UNIVERSITY OF NEW YORK AT STONY BROOK
DIRECTOR, MEDICAL INTENSIVE CARE UNIT
NASSAU COUNTY MEDICAL CENTER
EAST MEADOW, NEW YORK

FAROQUE A. KHAN, MB, MACP, FCCP, FRCP(C)

PROFESSOR OF MEDICINE
STATE UNIVERSITY OF NEW YORK AT STONY BROOK
CHAIRMAN, DEPARTMENT OF MEDICINE
NASSAU COUNTY MEDICAL CENTER
EAST MEADOW, NEW YORK

American College of Physicians
Philadelphia, Pennsylvania

Acquisitions Editor: Mary K. Ruff
Manager, Book Publishing: David Myers
Administrator, Book Publishing: Diane M. McCabe
Production Supervisor: Allan S. Kleinberg
Production Editor: Victoria Hoenigke
Cover Design: Barry Moshinski

American College of Physicians (ACP) became an imprint of the American College of Physicians–American Society of Internal Medicine in July 1998.

Printed in the United States of America.
Composition by CJS-Tapsco.
Printing/binding by Versa Press.

American College of Physicians–American Society of Internal Medicine
190 N. Independence Mall West
Philadelphia, PA 19106-1572

Library of Congress Cataloging-in-Publication Data

Mechanical ventilation manual/compiled and edited by Suhail Raoof,
　　Faroque A. Khan.
　　　　p.　cm.
　　　Includes bibliographical references.
　　　ISBN 0-943126-57-6 (alk. paper).
　　　1. Respirators—Handbooks, manuals, etc.　2. Respiratory therapy—Handbooks, manuals, etc.
　　I. Raoof, Suhail, 1961–　.　II. Khan, Faroque A.
　　　[DNLM:　1. Respiration, Artificial—methods—handbooks.
　　2. Ventilators, Mechanical—handbooks.　WF 39 M486 1997]
　　RC735.I5M45　　　1998
　　615.8′36—dc21
　　DNLM/DLC
　　for Library of Congress　　　　　　　　　　　　　　　　　　98-3305
　　　　　　　　　　　　　　　　　　　　　　　　　　　　　　　　　CIP

00 01 02 03 / 9 8 7 6 5 4 3 2

Acknowledgments

The authors wish to thank Dr. Ernesto Jonas for his invaluable suggestions and help in putting this book together. They would also like to acknowledge the hard work and remarkable computer graphic skills shown by Christina Esposito in the original typesetting, formatting, and designing of this handbook, including the diagrammatic representations.

CONTRIBUTORS

Suhail Allaqaband, MD
Pulmonary Research Fellow, Department
of Medicine, Nassau County Medical
Center
East Meadow, New York

**Christos P. Carvounis, MD, FACP,
FCCP, FACN**
Professor of Medicine, State University of
New York at Stony Brook
Stony Brook, New York
Chief, Division of Nephrology
Nassau County Medical Center
East Meadow, New York

Naseer Chowdhrey, MD
Pulmonary Research Fellow
Department of Medicine
Nassau County Medical Center
East Meadow, New York

Douglas Colquhoun, RRT
Associate Director, Respiratory Care
Nassau County Medical Center
East Meadow, New York

Liziamma George, MD
Assistant Professor of Medicine,
State University of New York
at Stony Brook
Stony Brook, New York

Rammohan Gumpeni, MD
Attending Physician
Patterson Geriatrics Center
Uniondale, New York

Robert M. Kacmarek, PhD
Associate Professor, Department of
Anesthesia
Harvard Medical School
Director, Respiratory Care
Massachusetts General Hospital
Boston, Massachusetts

**Ashok Karnik, MD, FRCP (London),
FCCP, FACP**
Associate Professor, State University of
New York at Stony Brook
Stony Brook, New York
Attending Physician, Division of Pulmonary
Diseases
Nassau County Medical Center
East Meadow, New York

**Faroque A. Khan, MB, MACP, FCCP,
FRCP(C)**
Professor of Medicine, State University of
New York at Stony Brook
Stony Brook, New York
Chairman, Department of Medicine
Nassau County Medical Center
East Meadow, New York

Raymond Lavery, RRT
Director, Respiratory Care
Nassau County Medical Center
East Meadow, New York

Younes Magdy, MD, PhD, FRCP(C)
Professor of Medicine
Section of Respiratory Diseases
University of Manitoba and Health
Science Center
Winnipeg, Manitoba

Maria Ninivaggi, RN, MSN, CIC
Assistant Director, Infection Control
Nassau County Medical Center
East Meadow, New York

Linga Raju, MD, FACP, FCCP
Associate Professor of Medicine,
State University of New York
at Stony Brook
Stony Brook, New York
Chief, Pulmonary Division
Nassau County Medical Center
East Meadow, New York

Suhail Raoof, MD, FACP, FCCP
Assistant Professor of Medicine,
State University of New York
at Stony Brook
Stony Brook, New York
Director, Medical Intensive Care Unit
Nassau County Medical Center
East Meadow, New York

Patricia Scrak, BBA
Director, Finance Office
A. Holly Patterson Division of Nassau
County Medical Center
East Meadow, New York

Joanne Selva, RN, BS, CIC
Director, Infection Control
Nassau County Medical Center
East Meadow, New York

PREFACE

Since 1988 I have been presenting workshops at the Annual Session of the American College of Physicians. Over the years, many of the workshop attendees have encouraged us to compile our material as a manual. In doing so, we have also incorporated into the manual many of the suggestions and critique offered by the attendees. We have attempted to keep the needs of the internists and house officers in mind, making liberal use of tables, simple graphs, figures, and algorithms in order to simplify the explanation of basic concepts. We have placed special emphasis on the newer advances in the rapidly expanding field of mechanical ventilation and, wherever possible, have used specific examples to make the connection between "theory" and "practice" more realistic.

We have also compiled the experience gained from the 11-bed medical intensive care unit and the 17-bed chronic ventilator ward at Nassau County Medical Center, New York, and presented it in the relevant sections.

This manual is *not* meant to be an exhaustive review of the subject; rather, it is designed to serve as a quick reference manual of the clinically important questions faced in starting patients on mechanical ventilation and, later, in weaning them from the ventilators.

This manual would not have been possible without the encouragement and support of the American College of Physicians staff and the contributors, all of whom were very generous with their advice and scholarly input. Thank you.

We hope that the *Mechanical Ventilation Manual* will meet the expectations of the readers, and we look forward to receiving your critiques.

Faroque A. Khan, MB, MACP, FCCP, FRCP(C)

CONTENTS

Part I. Why Ventilate?

1 Classification of Respiratory Failure   **1**
Faroque A. Khan, MB
Suhail Raoof, MD

Distinction between ventilatory and oxygenation failure is made. Various components of the respiratory system and examples of diseases that can affect them are discussed.

2 Indications for Ventilatory Support   **3**
Robert M. Kacmarek, PhD

Absolute and relative indications for the initiation of mechanical ventilation are outlined. Diseases generally requiring ventilatory support are listed.

3 Objectives of Mechanical Ventilation   **4**
Suhail Raoof, MD

The common reasons for mechanical ventilation are described.

Part II. How To Ventilate

4 Types of Ventilators   **7**
Robert M. Kacmarek, PhD

Discusses the two types of ventilators: negative- and positive-pressure ventilators. Advantages and disadvantages of negative-pressure ventilation and its clinical applications are discussed. Different types of positive-pressure ventilation are defined. Ventilators for in-hospital use, transport purposes, and home use are compared.

5 Pressure-Targeted Versus Volume-Targeted Ventilation and the Effects of Increasing Inspiratory Time   **11**
Robert M. Kacmarek, PhD

The differences between pressure- and volume-targeted ventilation are discussed.

6 Basics of Initial Ventilator Set-Up   **15**
Suhail Raoof, MD

Selection of appropriate tidal volume, rate, oxygen concentration, flow rate, and inspiratory flow pattern is discussed.

7 Modes of Ventilation   **21**
Suhail Raoof, MD

A description is given of different modes of mechanical ventilation (controlled mode, assist/control, synchronous intermittent mandatory ventilation, pressure support, and inverse ratio ventilation, mandatory minute ventilation, airway pressure release ventilation, proportional assist ventilation, and high-frequency ventilation). A brief summary of the advantages, disadvantages, indications, and principles of initial set-up of each mode is included.

8 Positive End-Expiratory Pressure (PEEP)   34
Suhail Raoof, MD

A brief description of PEEP therapy is given: its advantages, disadvantages, indications, and techniques.

9 Noninvasive Positive-Pressure Ventilation in Acute Respiratory Failure   37
Robert M. Kacmarek, PhD

This section encompasses the physiologic effects of noninvasive positive-pressure ventilation—its indications and contraindications, algorithmic approach, selection of masks, and compatible ventilator modes. A brief description of bilevel airway pressure ventilation is included.

10 Newer Techniques of Ventilation and Oxygenation   41
Liziamma George, MD

Conventional mechanical ventilation results in suboptimal distribution of gases and high pressures. Some new ventilator modes and techniques are enumerated. The advantages, disadvantages, and clinical applications of these techniques are discussed.

11 Airway Management   49
Suhail Raoof, MD

The advantages of orotracheal and nasotracheal intubations are enumerated. Commonly used sedatives and neuromuscular blocking agents, used for intubation and during mechanical ventilation, are described. Tracheostomy—its advantages and disadvantages—is also discussed.

12 Monitoring During Mechanical Ventilation   56
Suhail Raoof, MD

Special emphasis is given to the phenomenon of static and dynamic compliance and auto-PEEP. A simple technique of measuring compliance, using pressure volume curves, is discussed. The importance of auto-PEEP, including the method to measure it, and its effects are described. The influence of PEEP on pulmonary artery occlusion pressure is estimated.

13 Weaning from Mechanical Ventilation   69
Suhail Raoof, MD

Discusses nonpulmonary factors that need to be addressed before a patient is weaned from a ventilator. Weaning indices are described. Techniques of weaning include T-piece, IMV, and pressure support. A traditional extubation protocol is discussed, as are the post-extubation parameters. Finally, an algorithm for localizing the problem in the difficult-to-wean patient is included.

14 Terminal Withdrawal of Mechanical Ventilation from Patients in Persistent Vegetative State   86
Ashok Karnik, MD

The experience gained at Nassau County Medical Center, New York, with terminal weaning is discussed. A checklist of medico-legal issues and an algorithmic approach to terminal weaning are presented.

Part III. Problems During Mechanical Ventilation

15 Complications of Mechanical Ventilation   89
Suhail Allaqaband, MD

Limitations of conventional ventilation are described. Describes the commonly encountered complications during mechanical ventilation, with special emphasis on mechanical failure, barotrauma, nosocomial pneumonia, and oxygen toxicity.

16 Special Problems with Mechanical Ventilation in Different Clinical Settings   104
Suhail Raoof, MD

The physiologic basis of problems encountered in different clinical settings is discussed.

17 Troubleshooting on Mechanical Ventilation   109
Faroque A. Khan, MB
Suhail Raoof, MD

An algorithmic approach is given on what to do when a patient is fighting the ventilator or if the ventilator alarms go off. Causes of worsening oxygenation in the mechanically ventilated patient are listed.

18 Nutrition in Mechanically Ventilated Patients   112
Christos P. Carvounis, MD

Nutritional requirements may increase during stress. However, mechanical ventilation poses a specific problem during feeding of the patient. Malnutrition may impair host defenses and may make weaning more difficult. Nutritional status can be assessed by estimating the fat stores, muscle mass, or visceral proteins. The Harris-Benedict equation may be used to predict the resting energy requirements. Principles governing nutritional therapy are outlined.

19 Financial Aspects and Prognosis of Patients on Mechanical Ventilation   119
Suhail Raoof, MD
Naseer Chowdhrey, MD
Faroque A. Khan, MB

Different studies examining the financial aspects of providing ventilatory support are enumerated.

Part IV. Appendix

1 Basics of Ventilatory Support   131
Faroque A. Khan, MB
Suhail Raoof, MD

—Practical Guidelines for Assessment of Need for Mechanical Ventilation
—Clinical Guidelines for Mechanical Ventilation in Specific Conditions

2 Diagrammatic Representations   135
Douglas Colquhoun, RRT

—Waveform Analysis Curves
—Compliance
—Flow Rates and Inspiratory Time
—Positive End-Expiratory Pressure

3 Commonly Used Formulae   **147**
Douglas Colquhoun, RRT
Linga Raju, MD

4 Case Studies   **150**
Faroque A. Khan, MB
Suhail Raoof, MD

—Status Asthmaticus (Case 1)
—Chronic Obstructive Pulmonary Disease—Part I (Case 2)
—Adult Respiratory Distress Syndrome (Case 3)
—Chronic Obstructive Pulmonary Disease—Part II (Case 4)
—Left Ventricular Failure (Case 5)

5 Compliance Measurement Exercise   **157**
Faroque A. Kahn, MB
Suhail Raoof, MD

6 Quiz   **158**
Robert M. Kacmarek, PhD
Suhail Raoof, MD
Douglas Colquhoun, RRT
Raymond Lavery, RRT
Linga Raju, MD
Ashok Karnik, MD
Liziamma George, MD

Glossary   **164**

Annotated Bibliography   **167**

Index   **181**

I. WHY VENTILATE?

1. Classification of Respiratory Failure

Faroque A. Khan, MB, and Suhail Raoof, MD

Figure 1

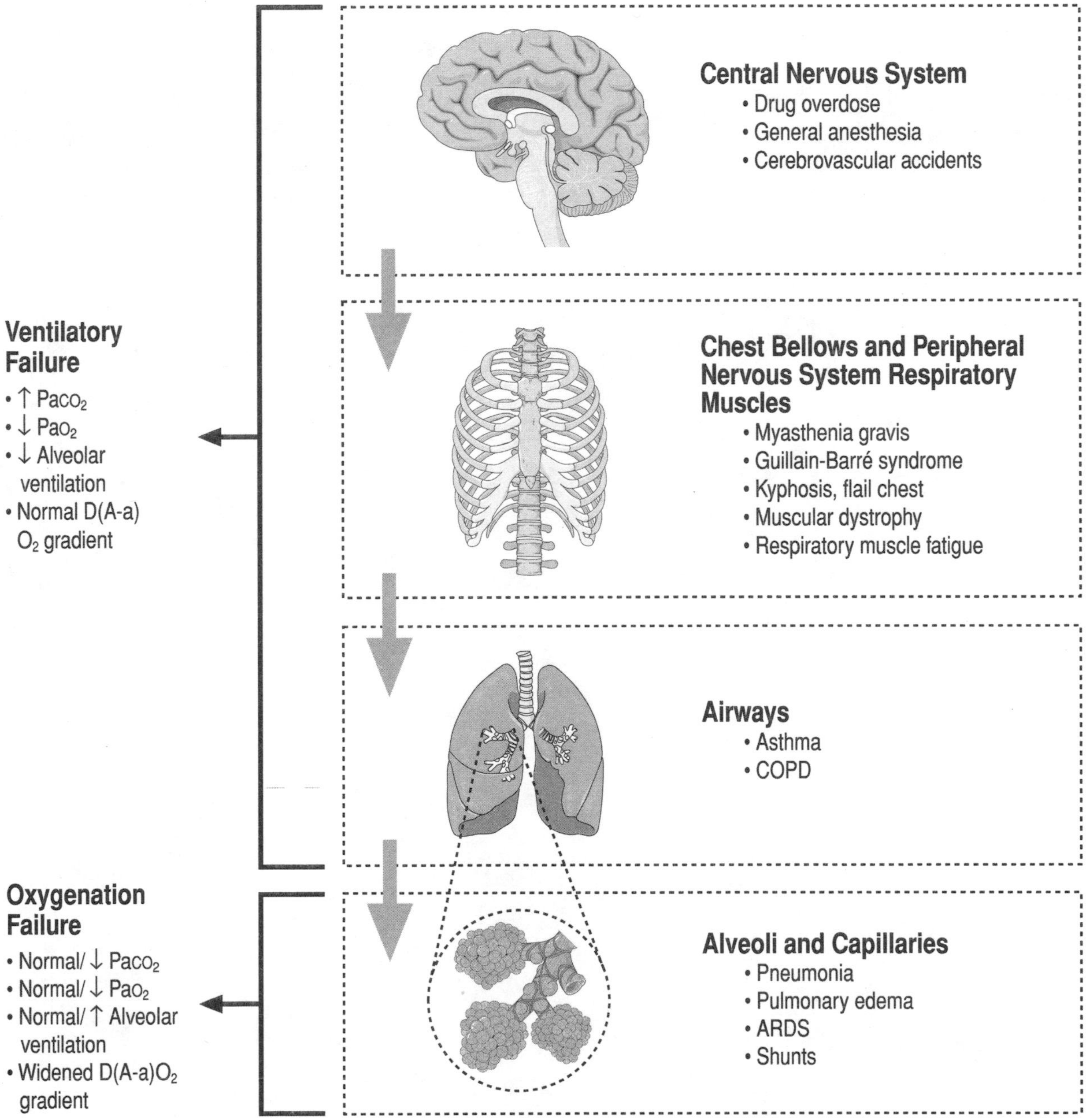

Ventilatory Failure

- $\uparrow PaCO_2$
- $\downarrow PaO_2$
- $\downarrow$ Alveolar ventilation
- Normal D(A-a) O_2 gradient

Central Nervous System
- Drug overdose
- General anesthesia
- Cerebrovascular accidents

Chest Bellows and Peripheral Nervous System Respiratory Muscles
- Myasthenia gravis
- Guillain-Barré syndrome
- Kyphosis, flail chest
- Muscular dystrophy
- Respiratory muscle fatigue

Airways
- Asthma
- COPD

Oxygenation Failure

- Normal/$\downarrow PaCO_2$
- Normal/$\downarrow PaO_2$
- Normal/$\uparrow$ Alveolar ventilation
- Widened D(A-a)O_2 gradient

Alveoli and Capillaries
- Pneumonia
- Pulmonary edema
- ARDS
- Shunts

1

The components of the respiratory system are intricately linked with each other. The central nervous system innervates muscles of the thorax via the peripheral nervous system. Contraction of the inspiratory muscles causes movement of the chest bellows, which allows air to flow to the alveoli. Thus, appropriate alveolar and arterial PO_2 and PCO_2 levels are maintained. Impairment of any component of the respiratory system may result in respiratory failure.

2. Indications for Ventilatory Support

Robert M. Kacmarek, PhD

- **Global indications**
- **Clinical conditions requiring ventilatory support**

A. Global pathophysiologic indications

1. Apnea
2. Acute ventilatory failure
   a. $PaCO_2$ >50 mm Hg and pH <7.30
3. Impending acute ventilatory failure
   a. Gas exchange data trending to failure (i.e., $PaCO_2$ increasing, pH decreasing) despite treatment
4. Severe refractory hypoxemia
   a. PaO_2 ≤60 mm Hg (SaO_2 <90%)
   b. FIO_2 ≥60%
5. Clinical signs of severe respiratory failure
   a. Unconsciousness
   b. Obtundation
   c. Agonal breathing
   d. Rapid, shallow breathing
   e. Severe abdominal paradox

B. Common and important clinical conditions when need for ventilatory support is high

1. ARDS
2. Asthma
3. Acute exacerbation of COPD
4. Chest trauma
5. Post-cardiac/thoracic surgery
6. Drug overdose
7. Severe neurologic/neuromuscular dysfunction
8. Head trauma
9. Severe pneumonia
10. Sepsis

3. Objectives of Mechanical Ventilation

Suhail Raoof, MD

- **To overcome mechanical problems**
  Rest fatigued muscles
  Administer anesthetics and neuromuscular blockers
  Prevent or treat atelectasis
  Flail chest
  Bronchopleural fistula
- **To regulate gas exchange**
  $PaCO_2$
  PaO_2 and SaO_2
- **Increase lung volumes**
  End-inspiration
  End-exhalation

Modified with permission from Slutsky AS. Mechanical ventilation: ACCP Consensus Conference. Chest. 1993;104:1833-5.

A. To overcome mechanical problems

1. Unload (rest) fatigued or overloaded inspiratory muscles, or inspiratory muscles showing incipient fatigue
2. Allow neuromuscular blockers, general anesthesia, and, sometimes, anticonvulsants and sedatives to be administered
3. Increase lung volumes to prevent or treat atelectasis (as in postoperative states or those associated with alveolar instability)
4. Chest wall problems such as flail chest
5. Large bronchopleural fistula with inability to ventilate or oxygenate (independent lung ventilation—HFJV)

B. To regulate gas exchange

1. $PaCO_2$
   a. Normalize: e.g., as in muscle fatigue, neuromuscular disorders
   b. Lower $PaCO_2$ to levels below normal: to decrease intracranial pressure, to offset severe metabolic acidosis
   c. Keep $PaCO_2$ higher than normal: acute on chronic respiratory failure, permissive hypercapnia for any reason
2. PaO_2 and SaO_2
   a. Reverse hypoxemia: e.g., as in ARDS, pulmonary edema, severe or multilobar pneumonia, other diffuse interstitial or alveolar diseases. (Increase PaO_2 generally to achieve $SaO_2 \geq 87\%$.)

b. Lower myocardial oxygen consumption, especially in cardiogenic shock states. (Mechanical ventilation can reduce myocardial oxygen demands by reducing preload and afterload of left ventricle.)

C. To increase lung volumes

1. During end-inspiration. (Improvement in ventilation/perfusion relationship and decrease in intrapulmonary shunting may be seen in mechanically ventilated breaths.)
   a. Treat severe hypoxemic respiratory failure.
   b. Prevent or treat atelectasis.
2. During end-exhalation (PEEP therapy). (PEEP → ↑ FRC + shifting tidal breathing to a more optimal portion of the lung's volume-pressure curve.)
   a. ARDS
   b. Postoperative atelectasis
   c. Other conditions leading to alveolar collapse

II. How to Ventilate

4. Types of Ventilators

Robert M. Kacmarek, PhD

- **General categories**
  Positive-pressure ventilators
  Negative-pressure ventilators
- **Comparison of positive- and negative-pressure ventilators**
- **Site-specific ventilators**
  ICU
  Transport
  Home

A. General categories
1. Positive-pressure ventilators
   Lungs are distended by applying an intermittent positive pressure to the airways.
   Ventilators may be:
   a. Pressure targeted → Gas flows into the lungs until preset pressure limit is reached
   b. Volume targeted → Gas flows into the lungs until preset volume is delivered
   c. Time targeted → Gas flows into the lungs until preset inspiratory time is reached

Figure 2

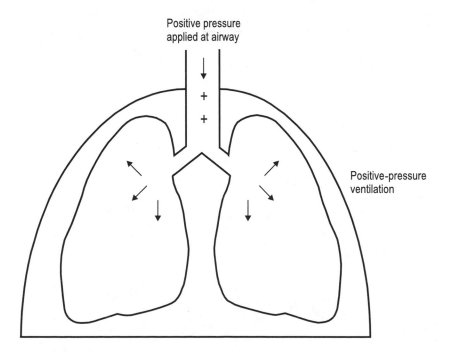

Positive pressure
applied at airway

Positive-pressure
ventilation

2. Negative-pressure ventilators
   The patient's chest wall is exposed to subatmospheric pressure during inspiration.

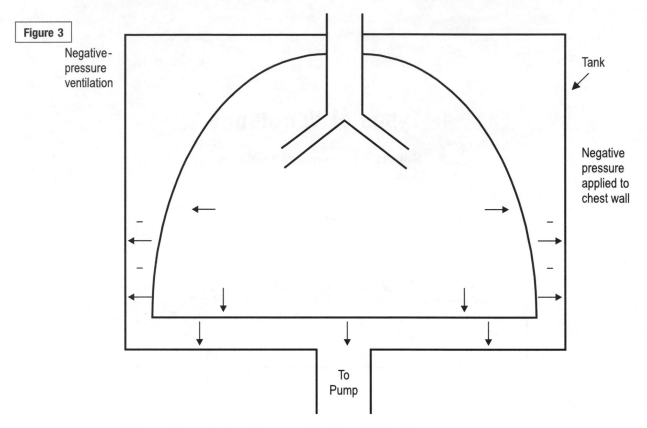

Figure 3

Negative-pressure ventilation

Tank

Negative pressure applied to chest wall

To Pump

B. Comparison of positive- and negative-pressure ventilators

	Positive Pressure	Negative Pressure
Overall versatility	High	Low
Ability to ventilate	High	Low
Invasiveness	High	Low
Mode variability	High	Low

C. Site-specific ventilators
   1. ICU
   2. Transport
   3. Home
      a. Volume targeted
      b. Pressure targeted

D. Comparison of site-specific ventilators

	ICU	Transport	Home care
Versatility of modes	High	Low	Moderate
F_{IO_2}	0.21–1.0	1.0 only	<0.4
Rate	Variable	Variable	Variable
Battery back-up	No	No	Yes
Patient monitoring	Yes	No	No
Patient system alarms	Extensive	None	Moderate or less
Overall adaptability	High	Low	Moderate
Availability of PEEP	All	None	Some

E. Suggestions for PEEP, CPAP, F_{IO_2}, and humidification system in site-specific ventilators

	Essential			Recommended			Optional		
	ICU	Transport	Home	ICU	Transport	Home	ICU	Transport	Home
F_{IO_2}	≤1.0	≤1.0	0.21	—	—	0.21–0.40	—	—	≥0.40
PEEP (cm H_2O)	≥30	≥30	No	—	—	No	—	—	≤10
CPAP (cm H_2O)	≥30	No	No	—	No	No	—	No	No
Humidifier	Yes	No	No	—	No	Yes	—	Yes	—

F. Modes of ventilation for ICU ventilators

	Essential	Recommended	Optional
Volume assist/control	Yes	—	—
Volume SIMV	Yes	—	—
Pressure support	Yes	—	—
Pressure assist/control	Yes	—	—
Pressure SIMV	Yes	—	—
Pressure or volume MMV	No	Yes	No
APRV	No	No	Yes
BiPAP	No	No	Yes

G. Modes of ventilation for transport and home care ventilators

	Essential		Recommended		Optional	
	Transport	Home	Transport	Home	Transport	Home
Volume assist/control	Yes	Yes	Yes	Yes	Yes	Yes
Volume SIMV	No	No	No	No	No	No
Pressure support	No	No	No	No	No	No
BiPAP	No	No	No	Yes	No	Yes
Pressure control	No	No	No	No	No	Yes
Pressure or volume MMV	No	No	No	No	No	No
APRV	No	No	No	No	No	No

H. Home care ventilators

	Pressure Cycled	Volume Cycled
Internal battery	No	Yes
Alarm capability	Low	High
Patient triggering effort	Low	High
Ventilatory target	Low pressure	Pressure and volume
Portability	High	High
F_{IO_2} variability	Low	Low
Overall popularity	High	Low
Patient-vent synchrony	High	Low

5. Pressure-Targeted Versus Volume-Targeted Ventilation and the Effects of Increasing Inspiratory Time

Robert M. Kacmarek, PhD

> - **Definitions**
> - **Comparison of volume- and pressure-targeted ventilation**
> - **Variables specified**
> - **Alteration of tidal volume, oxygenation, inspiratory time**

A. Volume-targeted ventilation: All modes are designed to ensure a constant tidal volume delivery regardless of peak airway and alveolar pressure.

B. Pressure-targeted ventilation: All modes are designed to ensure a constant peak airway and alveolar pressure regardless of tidal volume delivery.

C. Comparison of volume-targeted and pressure-targeted ventilation

	Volume-targeted	Pressure-targeted
Rate	Set or variable	Set or variable
V_T	Set	Variable
Peak alveolar pressure	Variable	Set
Peak airway pressure	Variable	Set
Peak flow	Set	Variable
Flow wave	Set, but variable	Set
Inspiratory time	Variable	Variable
I:E ratio	Variable	Variable

D. Waveforms: Pressure-targeted versus volume-targeted ventilation

Figure 4

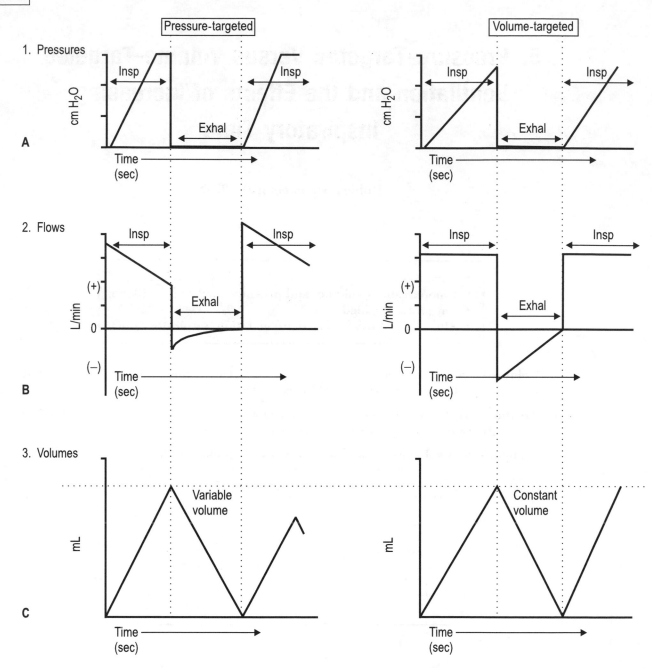

E. Available modes of ventilation

	Pressure-targeted	Volume-targeted
Assist	Yes	Yes
Assist/control	Yes	Yes
Control	Yes	Yes
SIMV	Yes	Yes
APRV	Yes	No
BiPAP	Yes	No

F. **Variables set during volume-targeted ventilation**
   1. VT or V̇E
   2. Rate or I:E ratio
   3. Inspiratory time or peak flow
   4. Waveform
   5. PEEP
   6. Sensitivity

G. **Variables set during pressure-targeted ventilation**
   1. Pressure levels
   2. Rate
   3. Inspiratory time or I:E ratio
   4. PEEP
   5. Sensitivity

H. **Factors affecting tidal volume during pressure-targeted ventilation**
   1. Inspiratory time
   2. Rate
   3. Set pressure level
   4. Applied PEEP level
   5. Auto-PEEP present

I. **Similarities between volume-targeted and pressure-targeted ventilation**
   1. Volume-targeted, decelerating flow with end-inspiratory plateau time, when carefully set, is indistinguishable from pressure-targeted ventilation
   2. Both decelerate flow over time
   3. Both deliver VT early in inspiratory pause time

J. **Clinical comparison of volume-targeted and pressure-targeted ventilation**
   1. Neither pressure control nor volume control has demonstrated a distinct advantage regarding
      a. Gas exchange
      b. Hemodynamics
      c. Pulmonary mechanics
   2. The primary advantage of pressure-targeted ventilation is its ability to target peak alveolar pressure and to automatically decrease tidal volume delivery when impedance to ventilation increases.
   3. Pressure control ventilation may more appropriately provide the high inspiratory flow demands of some critically ill patients (sometimes >120 L/min) compared with volume control ventilation.
   4. The primary advantage of volume-targeted ventilation is its ability to maintain a constant tidal volume delivery and to adjust airway and alveolar pressure automatically to ensure tidal volume delivery as impedance changes.

K. **Oxygenation status is dependent on:**
   1. Pathophysiology of the lung
   2. Oxygen-carrying capacity
   3. Cardiovascular function
   4. Peripheral tissue utilization
   5. FIO$_2$
   6. PEEP
   7. Inspiratory time

L. **Steps in the management of oxygenation in ARDS**
1. Optimize ventilation.
2. In the case of severe hypoxemia, adjust F_{IO_2} up to 1.0.
3. Adjust PEEP to above lower inflection point on P-V curve.
4. If adequate oxygenation is achieved, try to reduce F_{IO_2} to 0.8.
5. Increase inspiratory time; do not cause auto-PEEP to develop.
6. If adequate oxygenation is still maintained, adjust F_{IO_2} to 0.60.
7. Increase PEEP; avoid exceeding an end-inspiratory plateau pressure of 35 cm H_2O.

M. **Effects of increasing inspiratory time**
1. Increases $\overline{Paw}$
2. May recruit lung units with long respiratory time constants

N. **Avoiding the development of auto-PEEP when increasing inspiratory time**
1. Auto-PEEP develops in local lung units as a result of
   a. Lung unit compliance
   b. Increasing lung unit resistance
   c. Shortened expiratory time
   d. Increased $\dot{V}_E$
2. In heterogeneous lung injury at given ventilator settings, auto-PEEP will vary from one lung unit to another.
   a. Auto-PEEP is most likely to develop in high-compliance, high-resistance lung units.
   b. Auto-PEEP is least likely to develop in low-compliance, low-resistance lung units.
   c. In ARDS patients ventilated with long inspiratory times, auto-PEEP tends to develop in lung units where PEEP is least desired (high compliance, high resistance), resulting in over-distention.
   d. In stiff lung units in ARDS patients, auto-PEEP may not develop.
   e. Overall, auto-PEEP may result in maldistribution of local lung units.

6. Basics of Initial Ventilator Set-Up

Suhail Raoof, MD

- **Tidal volume**
- **Respiratory rate**
- **Oxygen concentration**
- **Inspiratory flow rate**
- **Inspiratory flow profiles**
- **Trigger sensitivity**

A. **Tidal volume (V_T)**
1. Tidal volume should be set for individual patient at 5–12 mL/kg of body weight (in volume-targeted ventilation).
2. Selected V_T may be influenced by respiratory system compliance, resistance, PaO_2, $PaCO_2$, and airway pressures.
3. If V_T is too low, atelectasis, hypoxemia, and hypoventilation can occur.
4. If V_T is too high, barotrauma, respiratory alkalosis, and decreased cardiac output can occur. (There is compelling evidence that the lower range of V_T limits stretch-induced parenchymal injury.)
5. The difference between ventilator-prescribed V_T and expiratory volume gives an indication of
   a. Circuit leaks
   b. Size of bronchopleural fistula
6. Proposed algorithm:
   Initiate mechanical ventilation with V_T of 10–12 mL/kg body weight
   ↓
   Stabilize patient
   ↓
   Lower V_T to 5–10 mL/kg body weight to:
   - To lower plateau pressure to ≤35 cm H_2O
   - To limit volutrauma

B. **Respiratory rate**
1. Usually started at 8–14 breaths/min if patient is otherwise clinically stable.
2. Higher rates may be necessary in restrictive lung disease.
3. Lower rates (limiting $\dot{V}_E$) may be important in a patient with chronic respiratory acidosis or for using the strategy of controlled hypoventilation.
4. If rates are too high, respiratory alkalosis, auto-PEEP, and barotrauma may occur.
5. If rates are too low, hypoventilation, hypoxemia, and patient discomfort owing to increased work of breathing may occur.

C. Oxygen concentration

1. If patient is hypoxemic, start at FIO_2 of 1.0. Brief periods of exposure to high oxygen concentrations are less detrimental than hypoxemic episodes.
2. Adjust according to arterial blood gases within 20–30 min to keep PaO_2 >60 mm Hg and thus keep SaO_2 >90%.
3. Sometimes in severe hypoxemic respiratory failure associated with elevated plateau pressures, SaO_2 between 87% and 90% may be acceptable. In such a setting, the oxygen transport may need to be optimized.

D. Inspiratory flow rate

1. Usually set at 40–100 L/min in volume-targeted ventilation.
2. Can increase flow rate up to 90–100 L/min in patients with high inspiratory demands. This may decrease inspiratory work, improve patient comfort, and decrease auto-PEEP. However, this also results in increased PIP.
3. Lower flow rates can be used to decrease the PIP and risk of barotrauma in patients with high initial PIP. This decreases expiratory time, however, and may lead to air trapping and patient discomfort.
4. Diagrammatic representation of flows.

E. Effect of inspiratory flows

1. Effect of inspiratory flows on the inspiratory time in mechanically ventilated patients

Figure 5

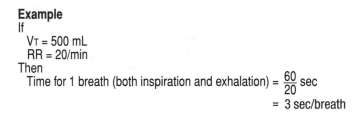

Example

If
V_T = 500 mL
RR = 20/min

Then
Time for 1 breath (both inspiration and exhalation) = $\frac{60}{20}$ sec

= 3 sec/breath

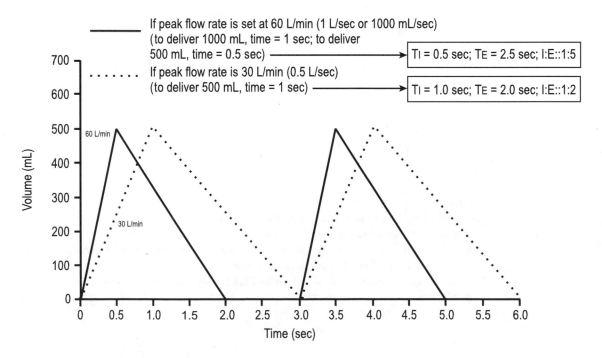

If peak flow rate is set at 60 L/min (1 L/sec or 1000 mL/sec) (to deliver 1000 mL, time = 1 sec; to deliver 500 mL, time = 0.5 sec) ⟶ T_I = 0.5 sec; T_E = 2.5 sec; I:E::1:5

If peak flow rate is 30 L/min (0.5 L/sec) (to deliver 500 mL, time = 1 sec) ⟶ T_I = 1.0 sec; T_E = 2.0 sec; I:E::1:2

2. Effect of inspiratory flows on PIP (illustrative values chosen)

Figure 6

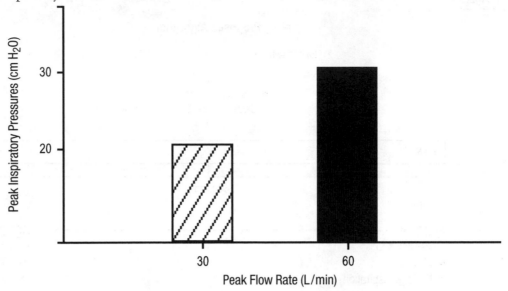

Figure 7

Proposed Algorithm

Begin with Inspiratory Flow Rate of 60 L/min

↓

- Stabilize patient
- Sedate patient if clinically indicated

Low		High

60 L/min

40 L/min   90 L/min

ARDS ←————————————————————————————————————→ COPD

ARDS
Lower flows to:
- ↓PIP
- Prolong inspiration

COPD
Increase flows to:
- ↓TI
- Allow more TE
  (minimize auto-PEEP)

SPECIAL PROBLEMS ————————————————————————————————————

Low inspiratory flows
1. Machine-delivered flow rate may become less than
   patient's spontaneous inspiratory flows

   Detection
   - Patient fights the ventilator.
   - Patient becomes dyspneic and diaphoretic.
   - Pressure dial on ventilator swings back and forth.

High inspiratory flows
High peak pressures

↓

?Barotrauma

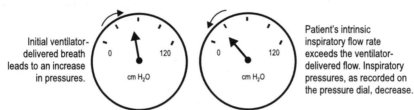

Initial ventilator-delivered breath leads to an increase in pressures.

Patient's intrinsic inspiratory flow rate exceeds the ventilator-delivered flow. Inspiratory pressures, as recorded on the pressure dial, decrease.

   Correction
   - Increase inspiratory flow rate to $4 \times \dot{V}E$ (e.g., if $\dot{V}E$ = 15 L,
     increase inspiratory flow rate to 15 × 4 = 60 L/min).
   - Sedate patient if clinically indicated.
   - Determine cause of increased inspiratory flow rate (e.g.,
     hypoxemia, low delivered $\dot{V}E$, CNS disorder). Correct if possible.
2. Development of auto-PEEP (longer inspiratory time; hence shorter
   expiratory time)
3. Delayed alveolar recruitment in the absence of sufficient PEEP

F. Inspiratory flow profile
  1. In volume-targeted ventilation, the following profiles may be available for selection:
     a. Constant (square or rectangular)
     b. Decelerating
     c. Accelerating
     d. Sinusoidal

Figure 8

Inspiratory Waveforms
(volume-cycled ventilation)

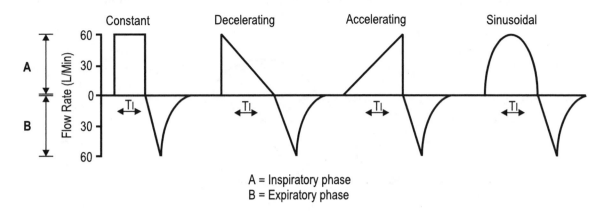

A = Inspiratory phase
B = Expiratory phase

2. Although the limited data available are conflicting, for clinical purposes no significant differences exist with the inspiratory flow profiles in terms of gas exchange or work of breathing.
3. The following theoretical considerations need to be made:
   a. Peak inspiratory flow rates remain similar for different flow patterns.
   b. The delivered VT, as expected, remains constant in all flow patterns with volume-cycled ventilation.
   c. The inspiratory time (TI) is longer with the decelerating, accelerating, and sinusoidal flow patterns than with the constant flow.
   d. Constant-flow waveform results in a higher peak airway pressure and a lower P̄aw. If one lung has lower compliance than the other, more even distribution of gases may take place with the constant-flow waveform (in contrast to decelerating flows, which may divert a larger portion of the VT to the normal lung).
   e. The decelerating flow results in a lower peak airway pressure, a higher P̄aw, and more rapid delivery of VT, which may promote early alveolar recruitment. If one lung has increased airway resistance, decelerating flow may result in more even distribution of gases.
   f. From a practical standpoint, a decelerating pattern may be beneficial in obstructive airways diseases and possible early, diffuse ARDS. If lobar atelectasis or other conditions with low and unequal compliance exist, a constant flow may result in better distribution of tidal ventilation.
4. In pressure-targeted ventilation, usually decelerating flow pattern with flow tapering determined by lung mechanics is seen. In patients with low resistance and low compliance, the inspiratory flow may cease well before the termination of the inspiratory phase.

G. Trigger sensitivity
1. Ventilator-trigger sensitivity is usually set at −0.5 to −1.5 cm H_2O.
2. Too sensitive: results in self-cycling.
3. Too insensitive: results in increased work of breathing.
4. *Practical Tip:* If the needle of the pressure dial shows a significant decrease in baseline pressure before the start of inspiration, the inspiratory trigger threshold may be too high (insensitive).

Figure 9

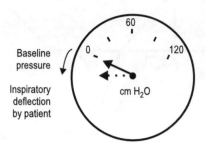

5. Flow-by
   a. Flow-by provides a predetermined flow of gas into the breathing circuit.
   b. The purpose of flow-by is to make inspiration easier for the patient by making the ventilator more sensitive to the patient's effort.
   c. Instead of the patient generating negative inspiratory pressure to trigger the ventilator, the patient's inspiratory flow will cause the flows to decrease. This results in triggering the ventilator and providing fresh gas to the breathing circuit. The delay in initiation of inspiration is minimized. Additionally, inertia of the demand system is obviated.
   d. Two flows are set:
      • Bias flow administered during exhalation.
      • Flow sensitivity, which, when reached, triggers the ventilator. (Triggering usually occurs when the difference between flow entering and exiting ventilator circuit equals a threshold value.)

7. Modes of Ventilation

Suhail Raoof, MD

> - **Controlled mode**
> - **Assist/control mode**
> - **Synchronous intermittent mandatory ventilation**
> - **Pressure support ventilation**
> - **Inverse ratio ventilation**
> - **Mandatory minute ventilation**
> - **Airway pressure release ventilation**
> - **Proportional assist ventilation**
> - **High-frequency ventilation**

Type	Description	Advantages	Disadvantages	Indications	Initial Setting
Controlled mode ventilation (CMV)	Ventilator delivers at a preset frequency. This may be pressure- or volume-targeted.	Guaranteed $\dot{V}_E$ or peak pressure	1. No patient interaction 2. Uncomfortable unless patient is comatose or paralyzed	Not used since advent of assist/control	Deliver adequate $\dot{V}_E$ (e.g., 10–12 mL/kg) or appropriate pressure $\times$ 10–12 breaths/min
Assist/control mode ventilation (A/C)	1. Ventilator delivers preset volume or pressure in response to patient-initiated breath. 2. A back-up rate is set to ensure a minimum respiratory rate.	1. Patient can increase $\dot{V}_E$ by increasing respiratory rate 2. Less work is required by patient to increase $\dot{V}_E$	1. Patient/ventilator dysynchrony 2. Respiratory alkalosis 3. Dynamic hyperinflation (air trapping) in COPD patients 4. Inspiratory muscle weakness	Preferred initial mode of mechanical ventilation in most situations	1. Deliver adequate $\dot{V}_E$ (e.g., 10–12 mL/kg) or appropriate pressure $\times$ 10–12 breaths/min 2. Sensitivity: −1 to −2 cm usually
Synchronized intermittent mandatory ventilation (SIMV)	May be pressure- or volume-targeted. Ventilator delivers synchronized breaths at preset V_T or pressure and rate, in addition to allowing patient to breathe spontaneously. Rate and V_T of spontaneous breaths are determined entirely by the patient. May be combined with pressure support during spontaneous breaths.	1. Decreased $\overline{Paw}$ (fewer complications) 2. Improved venous return (more physiologic) 3. Better intrapulmonary gas distribution possible	1. Less capable of changing $\dot{V}_E$ as needed 2. Work of breathing may be increased 3. Increased oxygen consumption 4. May prolong weaning (see Section 13E, p 79)	1. Primary means of ventilatory support, if adequate $\dot{V}_E$ is delivered 2. Severe respiratory alkalosis 3. To prevent auto-PEEP 4. Weaning method	1. Deliver adequate minute ventilation (e.g., 10–12 mL/kg) or appropriate pressure $\times$ 10–12 breaths/min 2. For weaning, initiate by supplying 80% $\dot{V}_E$ requirements from ventilator

(continues)

Figure 10

Modes of Ventilation

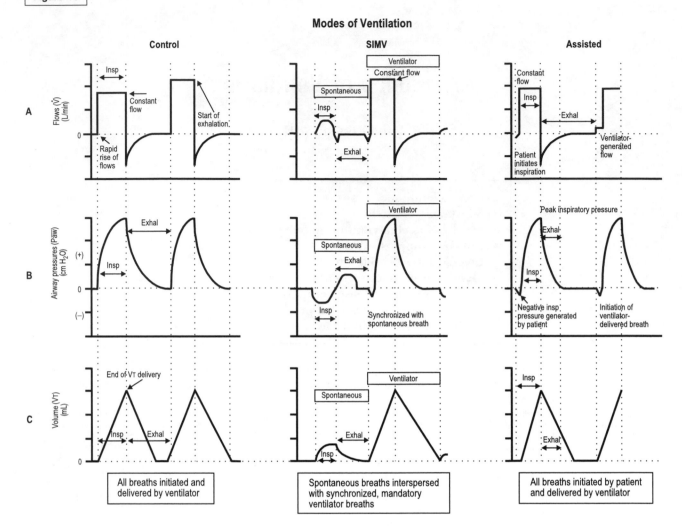

All breaths initiated and delivered by ventilator

Spontaneous breaths interspersed with synchronized, mandatory ventilator breaths

All breaths initiated by patient and delivered by ventilator

7. Modes of ventilation—cont'd

Type	Description	Advantages	Disadvantages	Indications	Initial Setting
Pressure support ventilation (PSV)	The ventilator delivers a predetermined level of positive pressure once the patient initiates a breath. Flow rate, inspiratory time, and frequency are determined by patient. A constant pressure is maintained until patient's inspiratory flow decreases to a specified level (e.g., 25% of peak flow value when exhalation occurs). (Crude analogy would be to compare the delivery of a spontaneous breath augmented with an Ambu bag.)	1. Partial ventilatory support may decrease inspiratory work of breathing. 2. Patient determines own inspiratory time, inspiratory flow rate, and V_T. 3. Improves patient comfort and reduces need for sedation. 4. Muscle reconditioning may be enhanced. 5. More rapid weaning may be possible	1. Unsuitable in absence of adequate spontaneous respiratory drive 2. Unsuitable with changing airways resistance (bronchospasm) and/or lung compliance 3. Doubtful efficacy in acute respiratory failure 4. Cannot use in-line nebulizers with flow rates exceeding patient's mean flow rate unless nebulizer is run by ventilator itself	1. Stable patients receiving long-term mechanical ventilation (to decrease amount of work of spontaneous breaths) 2. Weaning modality	1. Give enough pressure support to achieve spontaneous V_T of 10 mL/kg. Usual range is 10–20 cm H_2O pressure support. Gradually decrease over time to 5 cm H_2O, monitoring V_T and RR. At 5 cm H_2O, minimum PSV may be discontinued. 2. Minimum pressure support (L/sec) = $\dfrac{PIP - Pel}{\text{Peak inspiratory flow}}$ (Goal: To overcome airways resistance with PSV.)

(continues)

Figure 11

Pressure Support Ventilation

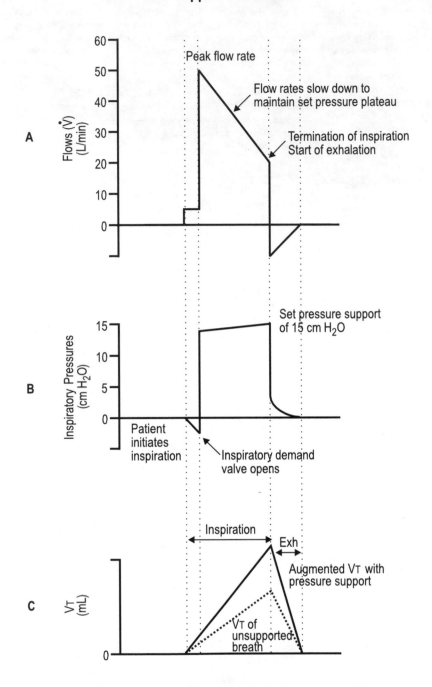

7. Modes of ventilation—cont'd

Type	Description	Advantages	Disadvantages	Indications	Initial Setting
Inverse ratio ventilation (IRV)	Prolongation of inspiratory time with proportionally shorter expiratory time (i.e., I:E >1) during CMV. May be applied with either pressure-targeted preset time-cycled (PCV-IRV) or volume-targeted ventilation (VCV-IRV). PCV-IRV: The inspiratory time or I:E ratio is set; inspiratory flow demonstrates a decelerating pattern. The V_T is variable. VCV-IRV: This is delivered by applying end-inspiratory pause or lowering inspiratory flow rate.	1. By prolonging inspiratory time, recruitment of lung units with decreased compliance or longer time constant is possible Collapsed alveoli ↓ Less ventilation ↓ Need sustained period of traction to make alveoli patent ↓ Prolong inspiratory time ↓ Recruitment of atelectatic alveoli ↓ Improved oxygenation 2. Maintains $\overline{Paw}$ at a relatively high level but keeps peak alveolar pressure within a safe range (as long as gas trapping does not occur) 3a. Volume-controlled IRV • More widely available option in ventilators • Allows delivery of preset tidal volume • Allows selection of inspiratory waveform 3b. Pressure-controlled IRV • Tighter control of peak airway pressure in inspiration • Improved tolerance by some patients	1. By decreasing the expiratory time, auto-PEEP may result (↓ BP, ↑PIP in VCV-IRV or ↓ V_T in PCV-IRV). 2. Barotrauma. 3. Sedation and sometimes paralysis may be needed. 4. Patient may need monitoring with a right heart catheter. (It is generally advisable to go up to I:E ratio of 2:1 but not beyond.) 5a. Volume-controlled IRV. • Peak airway pressures generally fluctuate. 5b. Pressure-controlled IRV. • Variable minute volume • Not available on all ventilators.	• ARDS with severe hypoxemic respiratory failure (especially with high FIO_2 requirements and PEEP). • No uniformly accepted criteria exist for initiation of IRV. Two proposed criteria are: 1. VCV-IRV FIO_2 >0.6 or PEEP >10 cm H_2O to maintain SaO_2 >90% 2. PCV-IRV Above parameters + PIP ≥45 cm H_2O	1. VCV-IRV. • Sedate ± paralyze. • Switch to decelerating flow pattern. • Keep V_T unchanged unless peak pressures >35 cm H_2O. If greater, lower tidal volume to achieve this target pressure. • Gradually reduce peak flow (from 60–80 to 40–60 L/min). • To prolong inspiratory time further, a 0.1–0.3 sec inspiratory pause may be introduced. • Add PEEP, if necessary. • Monitor vital signs, SaO_2 closely. 2. PCV-IRV. Similar to VCV-IRV, except set pressure limit (preferably up to 35 cm H_2O). This gets added on to PEEP (same or 50% of level of PEEP in conventional ventilation initially). Begin at 1:1 ratio, increase to 1.5:1, and finally to 2:1, if necessary. Monitor tidal volumes and pressure–volume curves. Avoid development of intrinsic PEEP closely.

(continues)

Figure 12

Inverse Ratio Ventilation

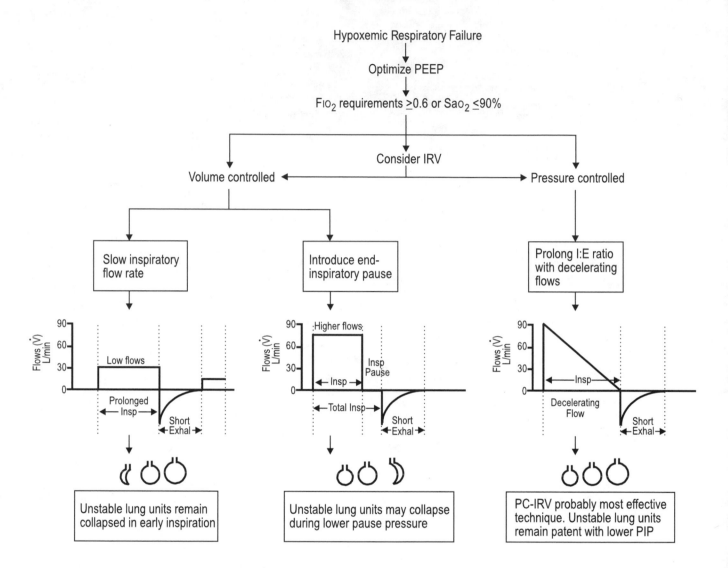

7. Modes of ventilation—cont'd

Type	Description	Advantages	Disadvantages	Indications	Initial Setting
Mandatory minute ventilation (MMV), also called extended mandatory minute ventilation or augmented minute volume	This mode guarantees that patient will receive a minimum, clinician-determined $\dot{V}E$. During this mode, if the patient breathes spontaneously, no ventilator breaths will be delivered as long as the spontaneous $\dot{V}E$ equals or exceeds the preset $\dot{V}E$. If spontaneous breaths are insufficient to maintain the preset $\dot{V}E$, ventilator breaths will be delivered to ensure that the sum of the mandatory and spontaneous breaths equals the preset $\dot{V}E$.	1. Ensures that patient's $\dot{V}E$ remains constant despite changes in ability to breathe spontaneously. 2. Prevents acute respiratory acidosis from hypoventilation or acute apnea. 3. Control of $PaCO_2$ is easier. 4. Transition between mechanical ventilation and spontaneous ventilation is theoretically easier. 5. Is less labor intensive.	1. Does not monitor alveolar ventilation (patients with rapid, shallow breathing may get an adequate $\dot{V}E$ but not an adequate V_A). 2. Minimum $\dot{V}E$ estimations are not well defined for patients. 3. Because clinicians need to make fewer ventilator adjustments with this mode, there may be less clinician supervision.	1. Drug overdose 2. Patients receiving intermittent heavy sedation 3. For patients with unstable ventilatory drive 4. Weaning mode (may be combined with pressure support)	1. Determine target $\dot{V}E$ (e.g., based upon projected $PaCO_2$, acid base status, stability of respiratory drive). For example, for weaning purposes, it may be set to 80% of $\dot{V}E$ on the assist control mode. 2. Set V_T to 7–10 mL/kg and rate to 8–10 breaths/min. 3. Titrate appropriate levels of CPAP, PEEP (if indicated), and FIO_2. 4. Monitor clinical status and ABGs and adjust appropriately.

(continues)

Figure 13

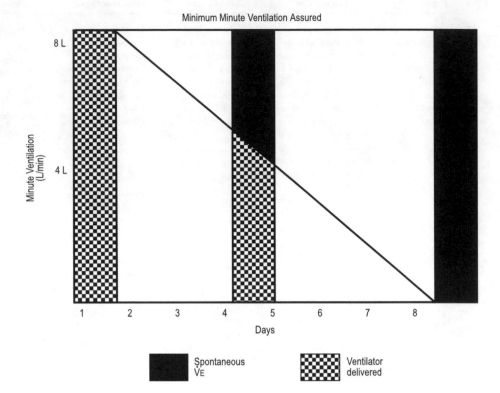

(Modified with permission from Thompson JD. Mandatory minute ventilation. In: Perel A, Stock MC, eds. Handbook of Mechanical Ventilatory Support. Williams and Wilkins, 1992:138.)

Mandatory Minute Ventilation

Minimum Minute Ventilation Assured

Minute Ventilation (L/min)

8 L

4 L

1 2 3 4 5 6 7 8

Days

■ Spontaneous V̇E

▦ Ventilator delivered

On Day 1, the ventilator is delivering the entire preset 8 L of V̇E. As the patient's spontaneous V̇E increases, the ventilator-delivered V̇E decreases until approximately Day 8, when the patient receives all of the V̇E spontaneously.

7. Modes of ventilation—cont'd

Type	Description	Advantages	Disadvantages	Indications	Initial Setting
Airway pressure release ventilation (APRV)	The ventilator in this mode will apply a supporting CPAP level and will augment alveolar ventilation by briefly "releasing" or decreasing airway pressure from the preset CPAP to a lower level. Lowering of CPAP level allows exhalation to occur. This mode was developed to provide ventilatory support to spontaneously breathing patients who have acute lung injury and who thus will benefit from CPAP therapy but need augmentation of alveolar ventilation. APRV uses intermittent decreases (rather than increases) in airway pressure to change lung volume. The V_T with this mode depends upon the pulmonary compliance and airway resistance, the extent and duration of airway pressure release.	1. Lowers peak airway pressures, hence minimizing risk of barotrauma. 2. Stabilizes collapsed alveoli by invoking intrinsic PEEP in some cases (due to short expiratory time). 3. Dead space ventilation may be reduced. 4. Allows spontaneous breathing. 5. May be delivered by face mask.	1. V_T (dependent upon airway pressure release) is influenced by compliance and resistance properties of the respiratory system. 2. Interference with spontaneous breathing (airway pressure release can occur during spontaneous inspiration)	Not clear 1. Mild acute lung injury 2. Alveolar hypoventilation states with minimal airflow obstruction	1. In patients with normal or mildly decreased lung-thoracic compliance: • CPAP: 10–15 cm H_2O • Releases: 0–2 cm H_2O • Expiratory time $\approx$ 1.5–2.0 sec • Inspiratory time $\approx$ 2.5 sec 2. In patients with moderately severe decrease in lung compliance: • CPAP: optimal level for best oxygenation • Release level: 5–10 cm H_2O • Expiratory time $\leq$ 1.5–2.0 sec • Inspiratory time $\approx$ 4.5 sec

(continues)

Figure 14

Airways Pressure Release Ventilation

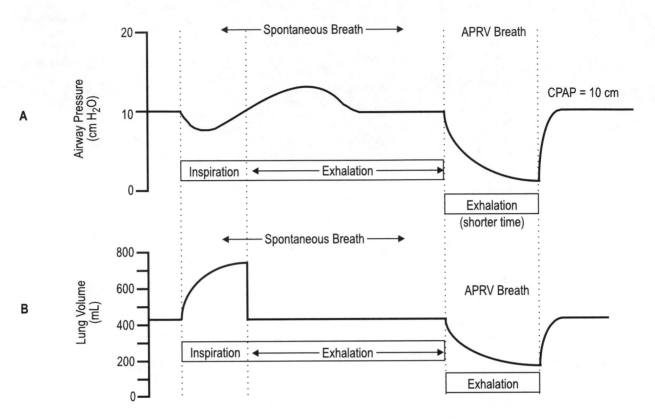

Modified with permission from Downs JB, Stock MC. Airway pressure release ventilation:
a new concept in ventilatory support. Crit Care Med. 1987; 15:459-61.

7. Modes of ventilation—cont'd

Type	Description	Advantages	Disadvantages	Indications	Initial Setting
Proportional assist ventilation (PAV) *S. Raoof, MD* *Y. Magdy, MD*	• The ventilator senses the patient's intrinsic effort to breathe ↓ • Ventilator generates proportional pressure and augments the patient's intrinsic effort. • The greater the patient effort, the greater the pressure the machine generates. • Delivered volume or pressure varies according to the input received from the ventilator due to the patient's inspiratory effort. • Determination of pattern of breathing is shifted to the patient.	1. Patient controls all the ventilatory variables (e.g., V_T, T_I, T_E, flow, airway pressure). Most physiologic mode of ventilation. 2. Easy to adjust on ventilator (only 1 variable is set, i.e., percentage of patient's elastance and resistance allocated to the ventilator). 3. Trigger sensitivity can be increased without significant artifactual triggering. 4. Lower peak airway pressures.	1. Air leak during inspiration leads to excessive "assist." 2. Air leak during expiration (with PEEP) may cause automatic cycling. 3. Occasional excessive "assist" by ventilator may occur. 4. Spontaneous respiratory drive is essential.	1. Stable mechanically ventilated patients (improves patient–ventilator synchrony) 2. Sepsis accompanied by hypotension 3. Noninvasive ventilation in short-term acute respiratory failure	1. Determine patient's elastance and resistance where total resistance = $\dfrac{\text{PIP} - \text{Pel}}{\text{Peak flow}}$. Patient's elastance: $\dfrac{\text{Pel} - \text{PEEP}}{V_T}$. 2. Set the ventilator's % assist to an appropriate level (approximately 80% of patient's elastance and resistance initially; less as condition improves) 3. Add PEEP if necessary. 4. Adjust peak pressure limit. 5. Adjust trigger sensitivity.

(continues)

Figure 15

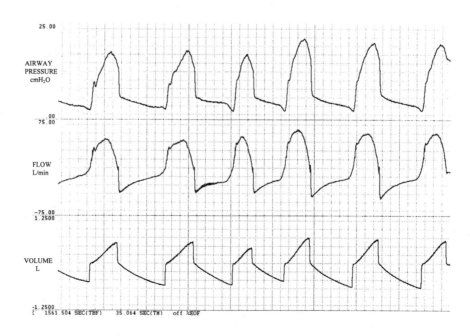

7. Modes of ventilation—cont'd

Type	Description	Advantages	Disadvantages	Indications	Initial Setting
High-frequency ventilation (HFV) 1. Applied at chest wall • High-frequency body surface oscillations 2. Applied at airway opening • High-frequency positive-pressure ventilation (HFPPV) • High-frequency jet ventilation (HFJV) • High-frequency oscillation (HFO)*	• The ventilator delivers small tidal volumes (1–3 mL/kg) at high frequencies (100–3000/min). • V_T delivered is less than V_D. Mechanisms of flow include: coaxial, Taylor dispersion, pendelluft and augmented molecular diffusion.	1. Potential for minimizing barotrauma (low V_T and thus low airway pressures) 2. Fewer alveolar pressure swings (less repetitive stretch) 3. Potential for improved ventilation perfusion matching (nonconventional air transport) 4. Some limited data that HFJV may be better than conventional mechanical ventilation in: • ARDS with circulatory shock • Low cardiac output states • Tracheomalacia • Bronchopleural fistula • Tracheoesophageal fistula	1. Contraindicated in asthma and COPD (risk of gas trapping) 2. Air trapping may occur in all patients 3. Severe necrotizing tracheobronchitis (inspired gases must be properly humidified) 4. Pressurized gas expanding in trachea causes significant cooling; heating device required 5. Outflow obstruction may lead to lung expansion and barotrauma 6. ?High gas flows may cause shearing in lung units with different impedance	1. Upper airways procedures; ENT surgeries, ± bronchoscopy (intubation is avoided with HFJV) 2. Thoracic surgery (e.g., descending aorta aneurysm resection) 3. To minimize movement in operative field • Lithotripsy (to minimize stone movement) due to ↓ respiratory excursions • Vocal cord operations 4. Bronchopleural fistula 5. Acute, severe respiratory failure in ARDS[†] 6. Patients at high risk for barotrauma owing to stiff lungs and high airway pressures (HFJV + conventional vent). 7. Patients in cardiogenic shock 8. Patients who cannot be intubated	HFJV[‡] • Driving pressure (DP): 25–35 psi • I:E::1.3–1.2 • Frequency ≈ 150/min • $FIO_2 = 1.0$ • PEEP = conventional ventilation ↓ ✓ ABG in 20 min

1. $PaCO_2$ inappropriate

To ↓$PaCO_2$	To ↑$PaCO_2$
• ↑DP	↓DP
• ↑I:E (up to 1:1)	↓I:E by 5% decrements until I:E::1:4
• ↑ f up to 250/min	↓f down to 100/min

2. PaO_2 inappropriate

To ↑PaO_2	To ↓PaO_2
—↑PEEP	↓PEEP
—↑DP by 5 psi increments (max. up to 50 psi)	↓FIO_2
—↑I:E	

---

*In a recent safety and efficacy study by Fort et al (Crit Care Med. 1997;25:937–47), high frequency oscillatory ventilation (HFO) was used in adults with acute respiratory distress syndrome. Seventeen adult patients who were failing conventional mechanical ventilation (including IRV) were recruited into the study. Their parameters recorded were

Variable	Mean	Range or SD
PIP (cm H_2O)	54.29	35–88
PEEP (cm H_2O)	18.24	7–34
Lung injury score	3.81	+0.23
PaO_2/FIO_2	18.33	+7.23
Oxygenation index	48.56	+15.17
($\overline{Paw}$ X FIO_2 X 100/PaO_2)		

Seventy-six percent (13/17) of the patients showed an improvement in their PaO_2/FIO_2 ratio and oxygenation index. Forty-seven percent (8/17) of the patients were weaned off HFO and put back on conventional ventilation. No deleterious effects on the cardiac output or tracheitis were observed with the use of HFO. This study used a lung volume recruitment strategy, which the previous HFV studies did not. Based on this small study, it appears that HFO may be a safe and effective way of ventilating adult patients with severe ARDS, who are failing conventional mechanical ventilation. Other studies are underway to answer this question.

[†] No data to demonstrate improved survival in such patients.

[‡] Adapted with permission from Standiford T, Morganroth ML. High-frequency ventilation. Chest. 1989; 96(6).

Description of High-Frequency Ventilation

Type	Delivery System	Freq (breaths/min)	V$_T$ (mL/kg)	I:E	Entrainment	Exhalation
HFPPV	Pneumatic valve	60–100	3–5	<0.3	(−)	Passive
HFJV	Gas jet <15–50 psi delivered via a 14–16 cannular gauge	100–600 (usually)	2–5	1:2 to 1:8	(+)	Passive
HFO	Oscillations generated by pistons pump microprocessors, etc.	300–3000 cycles/min	1–3	1:1	(+) Bias flow	Active

---

Figure 16

High-Frequency Ventilation

High-Frequency Jet Ventilation

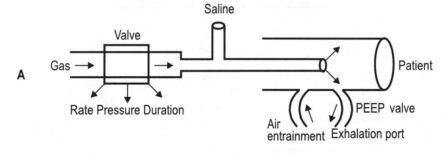

High-Frequency Oscillation

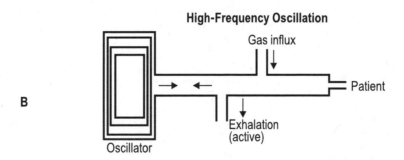

8. Positive End-Expiratory Pressure (PEEP)

Suhail Raoof, MD

> - **Description**
> - **Advantages**
> - **Disadvantages**
> - **Indications**
> - **Initial settings**
> - **Diagrammatic representation**

Description	Advantages	Disadvantages	Indications	Initial Setting
The ventilator applies a positive pressure at end-exhalation. Thus, supra-atmospheric pressure is maintained throughout the breathing cycle. When applied during spontaneous breathing, the term *CPAP* is used; when applied to a mechanically ventilated patient, the term *PEEP* is used; when applied at the end of exhalation, the term *end-expiratory positive airway pressure (EPAP)* is used. From a physiologic point of view, PEEP, CPAP, and EPAP are identical. Different acronyms are delivered from the controls of the equipment used to provide them.	1. Recruits and stabilizes collapsed alveoli 2. Increases FRC and prevents expiratory collapse 3. Improves oxygenation and lung compliance in conditions associated with diffuse alveolar collapse and hypoxemia 4. Used to decrease inspiratory work of breathing with auto-PEEP (see pp 64–66 on auto-PEEP) 5. May decrease lung injury and edema by maintaining minimum lung volume (minimizes shear forces associated with repetitive collapse and recruitment of injured alveoli)	1. Can impair cardiac output 2. Increases risk of barotrauma, esp. >15 cm H_2O 3. Increases intracranial pressure 4. Decreases renal and portal blood flow 5. Can complicate data collection in patients with right-heart catheters 6. Increases extravascular lung water 7. Increases dead space, if excessive 8. May increase inspiratory work of breathing, if over-distention occurs	1. Hypoxia with F_{IO_2} >0.50 in patients with diffuse bilateral infiltrates (e.g., ARDS, pulmonary edema) 2. Cardiac surgery to prevent postoperative mediastinal bleeding 3. Postoperative atelectasis (±)	**Technique 1** Begin PEEP at about 5 cm or 15 cm H_2O and increase or decrease in steps of 2 cm H_2O until optimal PEEP is achieved—i.e., - PaO_2 >60 mm Hg, F_{IO_2} <0.50, and hemodynamic stability - Achieving maximum static compliance of lung (Figure 17A) - Intrapulmonary shunt fraction <15% - Maximum $\dot{V}O_2$ **Technique 2***

* Technique 2 (supersyringe technique):
a. Sedate ± paralyze patient. Patient should not be making any respiratory excursions.
b. Suction respiratory secretions.
c. Ensure tight endotracheal tube/tracheostomy tube cuff seal.
d. Increase F_{IO_2} to 1.0.
e. Deliver single breath via ventilator to make patient achieve projected TLC.
f. Disconnect patient from ventilator.
g. Allow patient to exhale to FRC.
h. Take a super-syringe (filled with 1.0 F_{IO_2}).
i. Inflate lungs with 100 mL of O_2 at a time. Pause for 2–3 seconds. Measure Pel.
j. Keep inflating with 100 mL of O_2 at each step until a volume of 25 mL/kg is injected or airway pressure of 35 cm H_2O is reached or SaO_2 starts falling below 87%.
k. An inflation curve plotting volume and pressure is obtained.
l. Best PEEP is determined to be a pressure slightly above the lower inflection point (See Fig. 18).

Figure 17

Continuous Positive Airway Pressure and Positive End-Expiratory Pressure

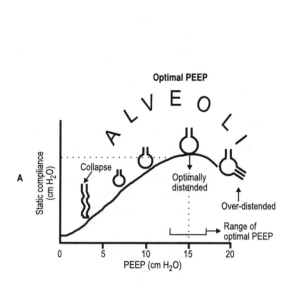

Optimal PEEP

A

Static compliance (cm H$_2$O)

Collapse
Optimally distended
Over-distended
Range of optimal PEEP

PEEP (cm H$_2$O)

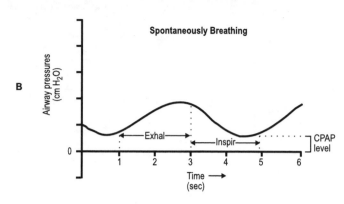

Spontaneously Breathing

B

Airway pressures (cm H$_2$O)

Exhal
Inspir
CPAP level

Time (sec)

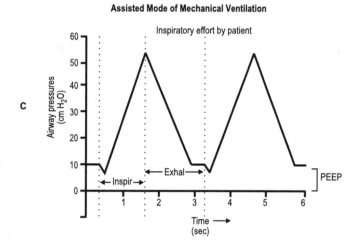

Assisted Mode of Mechanical Ventilation

Inspiratory effort by patient

C

Airway pressures (cm H$_2$O)

Inspir
Exhal
PEEP

Time (sec)

Figure 18

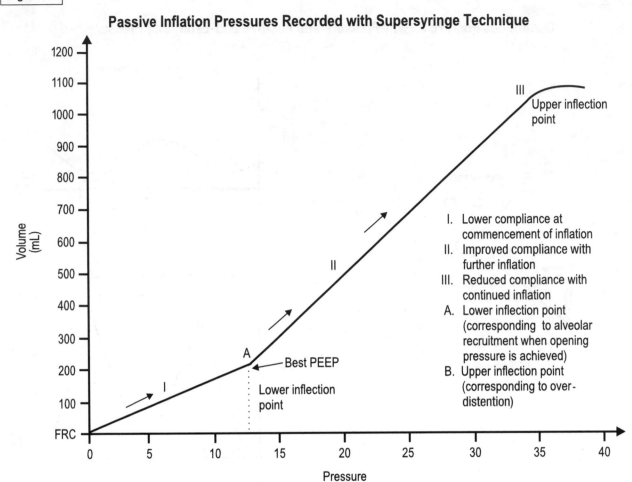

Passive Inflation Pressures Recorded with Supersyringe Technique

I. Lower compliance at commencement of inflation
II. Improved compliance with further inflation
III. Reduced compliance with continued inflation
A. Lower inflection point (corresponding to alveolar recruitment when opening pressure is achieved)
B. Upper inflection point (corresponding to over-distention)

Range of operating pressures recommended:
• Minimum (PEEP) ≈ 14 cm H_2O
• Maximum (Pel) ≈ 34 cm H_2O

9. Noninvasive Positive-Pressure Ventilation in Acute Respiratory Failure

Robert M. Kacmarek, PhD

- Physiologic effects
- Indications
- Relative contraindications
- Algorithm: acute COPD
- Initiation: acute respiratory failure
- Patient–ventilator interface
- Sizing of masks
- Type of ventilator
- Ventilator modes
- Ventilator settings
- Algorithmic approach—acute settings
- Bilevel pressure ventilators (BiPAP)

A. **Physiologic effects**
   1. Decreased diaphragmatic EMG activity
   2. Decreased accessory muscle EMG activity
   3. Decreased work of breathing
   4. Decreased transdiaphragmatic pressure
   5. Improved ventilatory pattern
      a. Elimination of abdominal paradox
      b. Elimination of accessory muscle use
   6. Improved gas exchange

B. **Indications**
   1. Hypoxemic respiratory failure, such as:
      a. Chronic obstructive pulmonary disease
      b. Asthma exacerbation
      c. Cardiogenic and noncardiogenic pulmonary edema
      d. Community-acquired pneumonia
      e. AIDS with disseminated pneumonia (e.g., *Pneumocystis carinii*)
      f. End-stage lung cancer
   2. Hypercapnic respiratory failure, such as:
      a. Chronic obstructive pulmonary disease
      b. Obesity hypoventilation
   3. Patients with acute respiratory failure who refuse intubation
   4. Postextubation in patients with marginal weaning criteria. NIPPV is also useful in transitioning difficult-to-wean patients from intubation to total spontaneous breathing.

C. **Relative contraindications**
   1. Respiratory arrest or need for immediate intubation
   2. Inability to protect airway/vomiting

3. Inability to clear secretions
4. Inability to cooperate or tolerate mask ventilation
5. Hypotension (systolic pressure <90 mm Hg)*
6. Uncontrolled arrhythmias*
7. Upper airway obstruction or facial trauma

D. Algorithm for ventilatory management of acute exacerbation of COPD

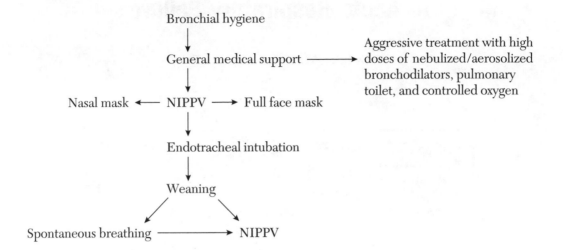

E. Initiation of NIPPV: Acute respiratory failure
1. Respiratory therapists and nurses should be supportive, encouraging, and attentive.
2. Available time: therapist needs to spend 60–90 minutes on initial set-up.
3. All aspects of NIPPV application should be negotiated with patient.
4. Patient needs to be involved in decisions regarding comfort and final pressure settings. A fully cooperative patient is necessary for successful application of NIPPV.

F. Patient–ventilator interface
1. Nasal mask
   a. Less claustrophobic
   b. Size critical for adequate fit
   c. Patient able to cough and speak
   d. Large air leaks likely without removing mask
   e. Normally less efficient ventilation than with full face mask
   f. Recommended for long-term use
   g. May be used for acute respiratory failure
2. Full face mask
   a. More claustrophobic
   b. Less air leak
   c. Size critical for adequate fit
   d. Must remove to expectorate and speak
   e. Better ventilation than with nasal mask
   f. Recommended for use in acute respiratory failure
   g. May be used for long-term application

* Hyptotension caused by auto-PEEP and arrhythmias caused by hypoxemia due to alveolar collapse may often improve after initiation of NIPPV.

G. Sizing of masks
  1. Nasal mask
     a. Small mask is always better than large mask
     b. Top of mask about one third of the way down from bridge of the nose; if high on bridge, air leaks into eyes
     c. Snug to lateral border of nose
     d. Resting above upper lip
  2. Full-face mask
     a. Small mask always better than large mask
     b. Top of mask about one third of the way down from bridge of the nose
     c. With most mask designs, lower border of mask rests just below lower lip

H. Type of ventilator
  1. Theoretically, any mechanical ventilator can be used
  2. ICU ventilator highly preferred over a portable, bilevel pressure ventilator because of:
     a. Accurate and consistent setting of F_{IO_2}
     b. Monitoring of patient rate, volume, inspiratory time, pressure, etc.
     c. Alarm package notifies practitioners of leaks, disconnection, etc.
  3. Portable, bilevel pressure ventilators recommended for long-term use

I. Ventilator modes
  1. ICU ventilators
     a. With a full-face mask
        i. PSV
        ii. Pressure assist/control (highly recommended)
        iii. Volume assist/control
     b. With a nasal mask
        i. Pressure assist/control (highly recommended)
        ii. Volume assist/control
        iii. PSV not recommended because termination of inspiration is flow dependent
  2. Portable pressure ventilators
     a. Pressure assist/control

J. Ventilator setting
  1. Do not exceed 20–25 cm H_2O PIP or gastric distention will become a major problem.
  2. Inspiratory pressure = 10–20 cm H_2O.
  3. PEEP = 0–8 cm H_2O
     a. Fluid status: initial hypotension
     b. Used to balance auto-PEEP
     c. Decrease work to trigger ventilator
  4. Use back-up rate so that during sleep, control ventilation is applied.
  5. V_T = 7–10 mL/kg.
  6. Always start with low pressure (5 cm H_2O) and increase as patient acclimates to positive pressure.

K. Applications of NIPPV in acute settings (proposed algorithm)

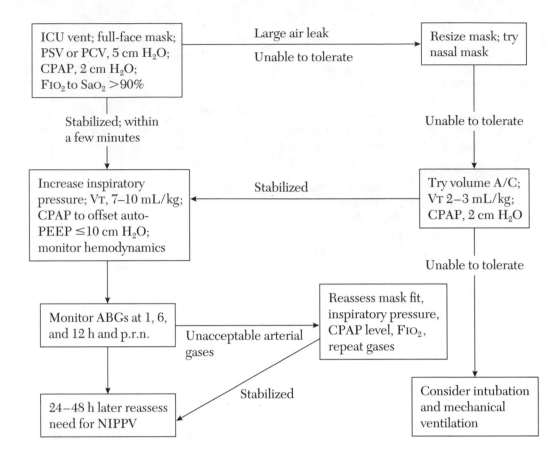

In the acutely ill, decompensating patient, a higher level of pressure support or pressure control and CPAP may be used initially or these pressures increased more rapidly.

L. Bilevel pressure ventilators, portable pressure ventilators
   1. Indications: chronic application of NIPPV
   2. Limitations in reference to application in acute respiratory failure
      a. Inability to precisely titrate high FIO_2
      b. Inability to measure delivered FIO_2
      c. Rebreathing of CO_2 within the circuit
      d. Lack of monitoring
      e. Lack of alarms
   3. Ventilator setting
      a. EPAP (CPAP) = 0–8 cm H_2O to offset increased triggered effort associated with auto-PEEP
      b. IPAP (pressure target) = 10–20 cm H_2O to provide effective ventilation
      c. Actual delivered V_T = 7–10 mL/kg
      d. Back-up assist rate set at baseline rate during sleep
   4. Patient–ventilator interface
      a. Nasal mask: preferred
      b. Nasal prongs: alternate
      c. Full-face mask: useful in some patients

10. Newer Techniques of Ventilation and Oxygenation

Liziamma George, MD

- **New developments in mechanical ventilation**
- **Limitations of newer techniques of ventilation**
- **Permissive hypercapnia**
- **Prone position ventilation**
- **New techniques useful in ventilation and oxygenation**

A. New developments in mechanical ventilation
   1. Ventilator modes
      a. Pressure-controlled ventilation
      b. Inverse ratio ventilation
      c. Airway pressure release ventilation
      d. Mandatory minute ventilation
      e. Proportional assist ventilation
   2. Ventilator techniques
      a. High-frequency ventilation
         i. Pressures applied to chest wall
            a) Body surface oscillation
         ii. Pressures applied to airway
            a) Passive exhalation
               - High-frequency positive pressure ventilation
               - High-frequency jet ventilation
            b) Active exhalation
               - High-frequency oscillation
      b. Decreased-frequency ventilation
         i. Permissive hypercapnia
         ii. Apneic oxygenation
         iii. Constant flow ventilation
         iv. Extracorporeal membrane oxygenation
         v. Extracorporeal CO_2 removal

B. Limitations of newer techniques of ventilation
   1. No randomized control studies available to compare with conventional mechanical ventilation
   2. Expensive

C. Permissive hypercapnia

S. Raoof, MD

1. Concept
   a. To achieve eucapnic state, high $\dot{V}_E$ may be necessary. This may result in:
      i. Elevated peak and plateau pressures
         (predisposing to volutrauma—especially in ARDS patients)
      ii. Auto-PEEP and dynamic hyperinflation
         (predisposing to volutrauma, hypotension, increased work of breathing—especially in patients with acute bronchospasm)
   b. Attempt to keep plateau pressures <35 cm H_2O and to prevent auto-PEEP from developing.
   c. Use low tidal volumes (5–7 mL/kg) in appropriate clinical settings.
2. Effects of using small tidal volumes

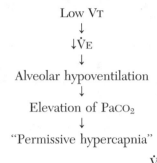

$$\text{Low } V_T$$
$$\downarrow$$
$$\downarrow \dot{V}_E$$
$$\downarrow$$
$$\text{Alveolar hypoventilation}$$
$$\downarrow$$
$$\text{Elevation of } Pa_{CO_2}$$
$$\downarrow$$
$$\text{"Permissive hypercapnia"}$$

$$\text{We know that } Pa_{CO_2} = K \times \frac{\dot{V}_{CO_2}}{\dot{V}_A}$$

where
$\dot{V}_{CO_2}$ = CO_2 production per minute, and
$\dot{V}_A$ = alveolar ventilation (per minute).

Thus, if $\dot{V}_A$ decreases, Pa_{CO_2} will increase.

3. Physiologic effects of hypercapnia
   a. Proportional reduction in Pa_{O_2} and hypoxia
   b. Rightward shift of hemoglobin dissociation curve (less oxygen binding with hemoglobin)—Bohr effect
   c. Vasodilation (except in pulmonary bed)
   d. Decreased cardiac contractility
   e. Hyperkalemia
   f. Inhibition of cellular enzymes
4. Clinical effects of hypercapnia
   a. Dyspnea
   b. Drowsiness
   c. Coma and narcosis
   d. Hypotension

5. Clinical example of permissive hypercapnia (80-kg patient with severe ARDS on mechanical ventilation)

	Arterial Blood Gases			
pH	PaCO$_2$ (mm Hg)	V$_T$ (mL)	Pel (cm H$_2$O)
7.36	38	800	55
	Lower V$_T$ to 600 mL		
7.28	50*	600	45
	Lower V$_T$ to 500 mL		
7.14	64	500	32
	Give IV HCO$_3$†		
7.23	66	500	32

* Allow PaCO$_2$ to increase gradually by 5–10 mm Hg per hour.

†No definite data on its usefulness exist.

6. Contraindications to permissive hypercapnia
    a. Raised intracranial pressure
    b. History of convulsions (may lower seizure threshold)
    c. Severe left ventricular failure
    d. Intractable or malignant arrhythmias
    e. Severe hyperkalemia

D. Prone position ventilation
Suhail Raoof, MD
1. Concept
    a. Dense consolidation of dependent (dorsal) lung units is common in ARDS patients who are kept supine.
    b. These lung units are richly perfused owing to gravitational forces.
    c. The net result is a shunt with refractory hypoxemia.
    d. By turning the patient in the prone position, theoretically the less consolidated areas will receive more ventilation and perfusion.
2. Mechanism
    a. In the prone position, the weight of the heart is on the sternum (rather than on the lungs, as in the supine position).
    b. This may cause the pleural pressure to be less positive in the dependent areas and hence decrease atelectasis of alveoli.
    c. Thus, there appears to be a more homogeneous distribution of regional ventilation in the prone position than in the supine position.
    d. Regional perfusion is relatively unaffected by changing from the supine to the prone position.
    e. The net effect is a reduction in the ventilation perfusion mismatching and improvement in oxygenation.

3. Effects of prone positioning in ARDS
   a. More than 60% of patients demonstrate improvement in oxygenation.
   b. The degree of improvement varies in different studies.

Author	n	Shows Improvement	Improvement in PaO_2 (mm Hg)	
			Mean Increase	Range
Douglas et al	6	5	69	2–178
Langer et al	13	8 (at 30 min)	20	12–32
Pappart et al	12	8 (after 20 min)	67	—

   c. Patients who benefit from prone positioning are likely to show some improvement in the first 30 minutes after switching from the supine position.
   d. The improvement in oxygenation is most likely in the early, exudative phase of ARDS.
   e. Improvement may be sustained in approximately 50% of patients even when they are switched back to the supine position.
4. Suggested technique:
   a. Sedation ± paralysis may be needed for some patients.
   b. ↑ FIO_2 to 1.0 approximately 15–20 minutes before repositioning.
   c. Ensure that patient is hemodynamically stable.
   d. Explain procedure to patient, if applicable.
   e. Use four people:
      • One person to stabilize endotracheal tube and ventilator tubing;
      • One person to stabilize vascular access, right heart catheter and arterial line, if applicable;
      • Two people to turn the patient from the supine to the lateral and finally the prone position.
   f. Do not apply pressure to the abdomen. The chest and pelvis should be supported during the turn.
   g. Support the head, chest, and pelvis with pillows. This should relieve the abdomen of most of the pressure that may otherwise be conferred by the weight of the patient in the supine position.
   h. The following parameters are checked:
      • PIPs (raised if ventilator tubing gets kinked in volume targeted ventilation)
      • V_T (lowered if either airways resistance is increased or chest wall compliance is decreased in pressure targeted ventilation)
      • SaO_2 (to ensure patient has not become hypoxemic)
   i. Suction the patient. (Repositioning may sometimes allow copious secretions and edema fluid to come into airways.)
   j. FIO_2 is lowered to prepositioning levels within 10–15 minutes.
   k. The patient is switched from prone to supine position (and from supine to prone) every 12 hours (most centers follow an 8- to 12-hour schedule). Patients who demonstrate a significant deterioration with prone positioning may be reverted back to supine position earlier.
5. Complications
   a. Dislodging endotracheal tubes, central and peripheral venous access lines, or arterial lines, urinary bladder catheters, etc.
   b. Hemodynamic instability or arrhythmias
   c. Worsening oxygenation
   d. Bed sores at pressure points
   e. Periorbital and conjunctival edema

E. New techniques useful in ventilation and oxygenation

Type	Description	Advantages	Disadvantages
Tracheal insufflation of oxygen (TRIO)	O_2 at a rate of 2–3 L is delivered to the lung through a catheter placed 1 cm proximal to the carina or deeper in the lung. Oxygenation is improved by turbulence of jet flow, cardiac oscillations and collateral ventilation and flushing of CO_2 from anatomic dead space.	• Useful in patients during surgical procedure on lung. • Adjunct to conventional ventilation. • Keeps the airway pressures to a minimum. • Useful as a temporary measure in difficult-to-intubate patients • Useful in patients who require continuous low-flow oxygen.	• Experimental in acute respiratory failure • If high flows are used, they may cause hyperinflation and volutrauma
Apneic oxygenation	100% O_2 is supplied via face mask or endotracheal tube to wash out nitrogen. $PaCO_2$ will increase at a rate of 3–6 mm Hg/min and PaO_2 will decrease by approximately the same amount.	Useful in assessing respiratory drive (spontaneous respiration).	• Prolonged respiratory support not possible • Maximum duration about 9 min • Indication—to assess brain death
Low-frequency positive-pressure ventilation and extracorporeal CO_2 removal (LFPPV–ECCO$_2$R)	Lung is ventilated using low ventilatory support. $PaCO_2$ is removed extracorporeally.	• Airway pressures are kept to a minimum and atelectasis of lung is prevented. • Exposure of blood to extracorporeal support is minimized, preserving lung blood flow.	• Bleeding may occur • Experimental in nature
Intravascular oxygenation	Bundle of microporous polypropylene hollow fibers is placed in the inferior vena cava. O_2 flows through the hollow fibers that will diffuse to the venous blood. That flow is between the fibers. Elimination of CO_2 is limited.	Improves oxygenation in selected patients.	• Diffusion limited gas exchange • Depends on gas flow cardiac output and hemoglobin concentration • Bleeding secondary to anticoagulants • Patient with small vena cava may not tolerate it, and surgical implantation may be needed • Experimental in nature
Extracorporeal membrane oxygenation (ECMO)	Salvage technique in patients with severe respiratory failure. Blood flows through artificial membranes outside the body. Oxygen is added and CO_2 removed. The access can be either venoarterial or venovenous.	Serves as a salvage procedure for severe ARDS patients.	• For adequate oxygenation, extracorporeal blood flow should equal cardiac output. • If venoarterial access is used, lung oligemia and subsequent lung necrosis may occur. • Additional positive-pressure ventilation is used to prevent lung atelectasis.
Extracorporeal CO_2 removal	By removing CO_2 extracorporeally, lung ventilation is decreased, resulting in lung rest. The CO_2 elimination can be achieved by 20%–30% of cardiac output flowing through the extracorporeal support using a venovenous access.	• Minimal ventilatory support, so ventilator-associated lung damage is minimized. • Maintenance of lung circulation, which will prevent lung oligemia and resultant necrosis.	• Bleeding • Experimental

(continues)

E. New techniques useful in ventilation and oxygenation—cont'd

Type	Description	Advantages	Disadvantages
Nitric oxide inhalation	Nitric oxide is a potent pulmonary vasodilator and can improve oxygenation and decrease pulmonary hypertension when administered directly to the lung.	• Nitric oxide is a potent pulmonary vasodilator. • The flow of nitric oxide to the lung units is proportional to ventilation. • Vasodilation occurs in ventilated lung units, leading to decreased ventilation perfusion mismatch. • The oxygenation improves and pulmonary hypertension decreases.	• Not FDA approved. • Nitric oxide is highly corrosive in high concentrations, especially in presence of moisture. • Rapid conversion to nitrogen dioxide in the presence of O_2. • Appropriate delivery and monitoring system is not available with adult ventilators. • Development of methemoglobinemia with prolonged administration. • Abrupt cessation leads to worsening hypoxemia. • Can cause increased LV preload in patients with pre-existing LVF. • Risk of atmospheric pollution in case of leakage.
Liquid ventilation (Perflubron) *S. Raoof, MD*	Perflubron is a chemically inert substance with a low surface tension and with high solubility for oxygen and carbon dioxide. Most clinical studies have used intratracheal instillation (via ET-tube or sideport) of perflubron approximately equal to the normal functional residual capacity of the patient's lungs—Partial Liquid Ventilation. This is done in conjunction with usual gas ventilation (commonly pressure-control ventilation) or ECMO. The usual indication is severe ARDS with hypoxemia.	May result in: • Significant improvement in oxygenation (opening of atelectatic alveoli, decreased $\dot{V}/\dot{Q}$ mismatch due to redistribution of blood flow) • Reduction in FIO_2 requirements (minimizing O_2 toxicity) • Increase in static and dynamic compliance—i.e., lower PIP and plateau pressures (reduction in surface tension at alveolar level), thus reducing barotrauma • ± Reduction of inflammatory response in ARDS • Reduced influx of proteinaceous and inflammatory edema fluid into the alveoli • Improved pulmonary lavage (inflammatory debris seen in ARDS floats on top of dense perflubron) • Greater cardiovascular stability due to success in reducing $\dot{V}E$	• Evaporative losses necessitate frequent restoration of desired perflubron volumes. • May occasionally cause mucus plugging of ET-tube. • During instillation of perflubron, some patients may transiently desaturate. • The liquid is radio-opaque and results in white-out of the lungs. • With pneumothorax, the liquid may come into the pleural space. • Certain plastic components of ET-tube, ventilators, or breathing circuits may get extracted with the solvent in perflubron.

Figure 19

Partial Liquid Ventilation (Gas and Liquid)

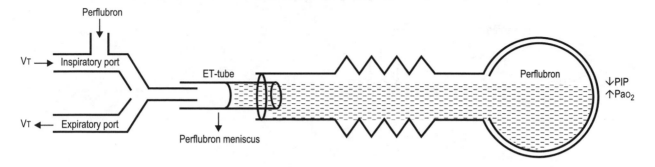

Figure 20

Intravascular Oxygenator

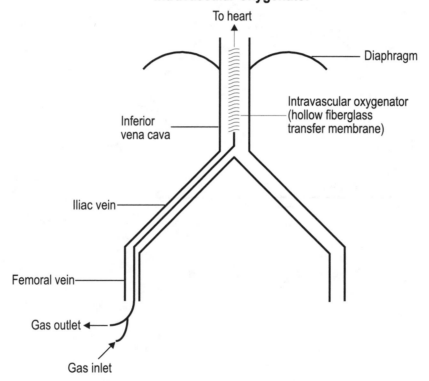

Figure 21

Venovenous Access for
Extracorporeal Membrane Oxygenation

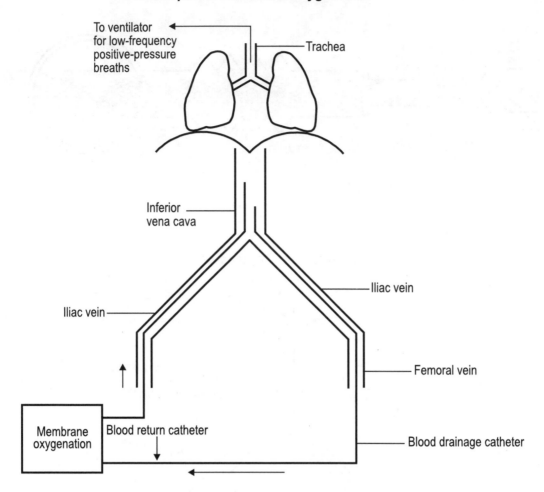

To ventilator for low-frequency positive-pressure breaths

Trachea

Inferior vena cava

Iliac vein

Iliac vein

Femoral vein

Membrane oxygenation

Blood return catheter

Blood drainage catheter

11. Airway Management

Suhail Raoof, MD

> - **Intubation**
> - **Commonly used medications**
> - **Tracheostomy**
> - **Airway cuff management**

A. Intubation

  1. Types of intubation
     a. Orotracheal
     b. Nasotracheal
  2. Features of each type of intubation

Features	Orotracheal	Nasotracheal
Advantages	1. Larger diameter tube can be passed that facilitates suctioning and bronchoscopy (greater than size 8) 2. Quick control of airway with direct visualization (useful in cardiac or respiratory arrest)	1. Better tolerated in awake patients 2. Minimizes sedation and paralysis 3. Better fixation of tube (more stable) 4. Fewer oropharyngeal secretions 5. Easy to perform: 92% success rate in patients without apnea
Contraindications and technical problems	Trismus, oral trauma, decerebrate rigidity, mandibular fracture, obstructing mouth lesions, temporomandibular joint disease, cervical spine disease	Nasal obstruction, paranasal sinus disease, otitis media, bleeding diathesis, lack of spontaneous breathing (technically difficult)
Specific complications	Oral, soft tissue and dental trauma, tracheolaryngeal injury	Epistaxis, paranasal sinusitis → bacteremia, dislodged adenoids, tube kinking, turbinate trauma, resistance (longer, narrower tube)
Indications	Patient with apnea During resuscitative efforts Bleeding diathesis	Awake, spontaneously breathing patient Acute cervical spine injury, facial trauma

  3. Indications
     a. Airway protection
     b. Maintenance of airway patency
     c. Pulmonary toilet
     d. Positive-pressure ventilation
     e. Adequate oxygenation
     f. PEEP
  4. Size and position of endotracheal tubes (for patients ≥ 14 years old)
     a. Internal diameter
        i. 7.0 ± 1 mm: women
        ii. 8.0 ± 1 mm: men

b. External diameter
　　　　i. 9.3–10 mm: women
　　　　ii. 10.7–11.3 mm: men
　　c. French units
　　　　i. 28–30: women
　　　　ii. 32–34: men
　　d. Distance from tip of tube
　　　　i. To lips (orotracheal): 20–24 cm
　　　　ii. To nares (nasotracheal): 23–27 cm
5. Airways resistance and ET-tubes
　　a. For laminar flow: resistance is inversely proportional to the fourth power of radius of the ET-tube.
　　b. For turbulent flow: resistance is inversely proportional to the fifth power of radius of the ET-tube.
　　c. Increase in airways resistance from a size 8 to size 7 ET-tube will be

$$\frac{(4)^{-5}}{(3.5)^{-5}} = 1.95 \text{ times}$$

　　d. An ET-tube as small as a size 6.5 mm may be inserted via the nasopharynx using low peak inspiratory flows (<30 L/min) without significantly increasing the airways resistance.

B. Commonly used medications (Society of Critical Care Medicine's Executive Committee Recommendations)

1. Analgesics

Drug	Drug of Choice	Advantages	Disadvantages	Half-life	Administration
Morphine	Analgesia (no amnestic properties)	1. Low cost 2. High potency* 3. Analgesic efficacy 4. ± Euphoria	1. Unpredictable effect (with dose) 2. Respiratory depression 3. Hypotension 4. Bronchospasm 5. Histamine release 6. Constipation 7. Urinary retention 8. Confusion	1.5–2.0 h	*Load*: 0.05 mg/kg over 5–15 min *Maintenance*: 4–6 mg/h or *Bolus*: 4–6 mg q1–2h
Fentanyl (Sublimaze) [synthetic opiate]	Use for analgesia in a patient with: • Morphine allergy • Histamine release with morphine • Hemodynamic instability	1. More potent 2. More liophilic (quicker onset of action) 3. No histaminic release 4. Less hypotension 5. No active metabolites	Accumulates in peripheral compartments (progressive increase in half-life, i.e., 9–16 h)	30–60 min	*Load*: 1–2 µg/kg *Maintenance*: 1–2 µg/kg/h
Hydromorphone (Dilaudid) [semisynthetic morphine derivative]	Alternative to morphine (10 mg morphine ~ 1.3 mg hydromorphone in analgesic effect)	1. Eight times more potent analgesic effect than morphine 2. More potent sedative effect 3. Less euphoria, hallucinations, muscle rigidity, tremors, and blurred vision compared with morphine	1. Similar to morphine 2. Must be used with caution in patients with severe COPD, suppressed respiratory drive, hypoxia, or hypercapnia 3. Must be used with caution in patients with head injury and increased intracranial tension		*Initial*: 0.5 mg IV slowly over 2–3 min *Maintenance*: 1–2 mg q1–2h ↑ by 0.5 mg usually

(continues)

1. Analgesics—cont'd

Drug	Drug of Choice	Advantages	Disadvantages	Half-life	Administration
Hydromorphone (Dilaudid) [semisynthetic morphine derivative]—cont'd			4. Highly concentrated formulation (HP) contains 10 mg hydromorphone per mL—needs to be used with caution 5. As with morphine, multiple drug interactions are possible (e.g., with other CNS depressants, sedatives, hypnotics, phenothiazines, tranquilizers, and alcohol)		

* Parenteral-oral conversion factor. Potency for equal parenteral dose relative to morphine is mentioned in parentheses: morphine sulfate 1:6 (1); hydromorphone 1:5 (6); codeine 1:1.5 (0.1); meperidine 1:4 (0.15); oxycodone 1:2 (1.0); methadone 1:2 (1.0).

Modified with permission from Shapiro BA, Warren J, Egol AB, et al. Basic parameters for intravenous analgesia and sedation for adult patients in the intensive care unit: an executive summary. Crit Care Med. 1995;23:1596-600.

2. Sedatives

Drug	Drug of Choice	Advantages	Disadvantages	Half-life	Administration
a. Midazolam (Versed)	Short-term sedation (<24 h)	1. Short duration of action 2. Onset rapid (2–2.5 min) 3. Anterograde amnesia	1. Prolonged effect with long-term use 2. Expensive	• Wide range (1.2–12.3 h) • May be prolonged in CHF	*Bolus*: 0.03 mg/kg *Maintenance*: 0.03 mg/kg/h
b. Propofol (Diprivan)	Short-term sedation (<24 h)	1. Sedative 2. Hypnotic 3. Anxiolytic 4. Anterograde amnesia 5. Onset rapid (1–2 min) 6. Effect rapidly reversible (10–15 min)	1. Long-term use: prolonged effect $t/2$ = 300–700 min 2. Cannot be used for intermittent IV administration 3. Preferably administered via central vein	• 5 min (after 1 h infusion of propofol) [clearance: 25–50 mL/kg/min in 70-kg adult]	*Initial infusion rate*: 0.5 mg/kg/h *Increase by*: 0.5 mg/kg q5–10 min *Usual maintenance infusion rate*: 0.5–3.0 mg/kg/h
c. Lorazepam (Ativan)	Prolonged anxiolytic use (>24 h)	1. Less lipophilic (less peripheral accumulation) 2. Longer acting (compared with midazolam) 3. Less hypotension 4. Less expensive 5. More rapid awakening after prolonged use	1. Delayed onset of action 2. Use midazolam or diazepam to initiate sedation (if rapid sedation is needed)	• 16 h (given IV)	*Infusion*: 1–4 mg/h usually

Agents not recommended:
- Etomidate (adrenocortical suppression ↑ mortality with long-term effect).
- Ketamine (↑ BP ↑ HR ↑ intracranial pressure).
- Diazepam (pain/thrombophlebitis at peripheral vein injection; dilution mandates large volumes of fluid administration; intermittent dosing regimen may lead to excessive sedation).

3. Neuromuscular blocking agents

Drug	Drug of Choice	Advantages	Disadvantages	Administration
a. Pancuronium (Pavulon)	Preferred agent	1. Inexpensive 2. Onset within 4 min	1. Long acting (75–90 min after one dose) 2. ↑ Histamine release 3. Mast cell degranulation (↓ BP, bronchospasm, ↑ HR, flushing) 4. ↑ HR ↑ BP (vagolytic properties) 5. Prolonged blockade reported (especially in conjunction with steroids)	*Bolus*: 0.06–0.08 mg/kg *Maintenance*: 0.02–0.03 mg/kg q1–2h or 0.02–0.03 mg/kg/h
b. Vecuronium (Norcuron)	Neuromuscular blockade for patients with: • Cardiac disease • Hemodynamic instability	1. Little or no cardiac effect 2. Rapid onset (2–3.5 min) 3. No bronchospasm 4. Shorter duration of blockade (25–30 min)	1. Liver metabolism 2. Kidney excretion 3. Expensive 4. Prolonged blockade reported (especially in conjunction with steroids)	*Bolus*: 0.08–0.10 mg/kg *Infusion*: 0.8–1.2 μg/kg/min

Reprinted with permission from Shapiro BA, Warren J, Egol AB, et al. Basic parameters for intravenous analgesia and sedation for adult patients in the intensive care unit: an executive summary. Crit Care Med. 1995;23:1596–600.

GUIDELINES FOR USE OF NEUROMUSCULAR BLOCKING AGENTS IN THE MEDICAL INTENSIVE CARE UNIT AT NASSAU COUNTY MEDICAL CENTER

Patient Requires Neuromuscular Blocking Agent

Patient with COPD or ARDS who has high PIPs; patient with status asthmaticus who cannot be ventilated; patient with status epilepticus who cannot be controlled with conventional medications

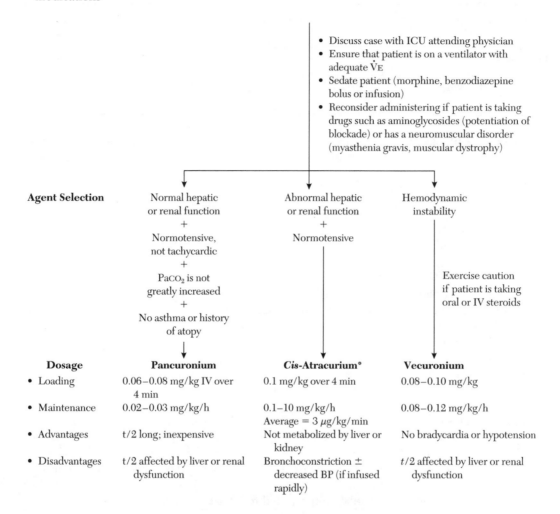

- Discuss case with ICU attending physician
- Ensure that patient is on a ventilator with adequate $\dot{V}_E$
- Sedate patient (morphine, benzodiazepine bolus or infusion)
- Reconsider administering if patient is taking drugs such as aminoglycosides (potentiation of blockade) or has a neuromuscular disorder (myasthenia gravis, muscular dystrophy)

Agent Selection

| | Normal hepatic or renal function + Normotensive, not tachycardic + PaCO₂ is not greatly increased + No asthma or history of atopy | Abnormal hepatic or renal function + Normotensive | Hemodynamic instability |

Exercise caution if patient is taking oral or IV steroids

Dosage	Pancuronium	Cis-Atracurium°	Vecuronium
• Loading	0.06–0.08 mg/kg IV over 4 min	0.1 mg/kg over 4 min	0.08–0.10 mg/kg
• Maintenance	0.02–0.03 mg/kg/h	0.1–10 mg/kg/h Average = 3 µg/kg/min	0.08–0.12 mg/kg/h
• Advantages	t/2 long; inexpensive	Not metabolized by liver or kidney	No bradycardia or hypotension
• Disadvantages	t/2 affected by liver or renal dysfunction	Bronchoconstriction ± decreased BP (if infused rapidly)	t/2 affected by liver or renal dysfunction

*Although not recommended by the Critical Care Medicine Society, we have been using *cis*-Atracurium in patients with moderate–severe hepatic or renal dysfunction or those taking systemic steroids.

Monitoring

(1) BP every hour and continuous ECG rhythym.
(2) Ensure that patient is sedated.
(3) Arterial blood gases at least q8h (if patient is stable) with continuous SaO₂ monitoring.
(4) Peripheral nerve stimulator: q4h (attempt preservation of one out of four twitches).[†]

[†] Using peripheral nerve stimulator to titrate dosage of neuromuscular blockers to abolish three of four twitches, Rudis and colleagues determined that the dosage of vecuronium needed was 0.04 mg/kg/h versus 0.07 mg/kg/h and that recovery from paralysis was significantly quicker in 50% of patients compared with those dosed by clinical assessment. (Reprinted with permission from Rudis MI, Sikora CA, Angus E, et al. A prospective, randomized, controlled evaluation of peripheral nerve stimulation versus standard clinical dosing of neuromuscular blocking agents in critically ill patients. Crit Care Med. 1997;25:575-83.)

Guidelines continue.

Discontinuation

All criteria should be fulfilled except in special circumstances (e.g., hemiplegia).

	Ready for Extubation	Keep Mechanically Ventilated
a. Nerve stimulator (q4h)	(+) Train of 4	<4 twitches
b. Hand grip (q24h)	Strong (5/5)	Weak (<5/5)
c. Head lift (q24h)	Sustained >5 sec.	Not sustained
d. PImax (q24h)	>-30 cm H_2O	<-20 cm H_2O
e. Vital capacity (q24h)	>1 L	<1 L
f. Discuss with attending physician (q24h)	Yes	No

Prolonged blockade   Reversal (Anesthesia Consult)

C. Tracheostomy
1. Indications
   a. Prolonged (usually >2 weeks) mechanical ventilation
   b. Relief of upper airway obstruction
   c. Laryngeal trauma
   d. Weaning patients with marginal pulmonary function
2. Advantages of tracheostomy over translaryngeal intubation
   a. Improved airway suctioning
   b. Improved patient comfort and mobility
   c. Decreased endolaryngeal damage
   d. Eating/speaking is possible
   e. Decreased airway resistance and work of breathing
   f. Safer tube changes (less chance of accidental extubation)
3. Disadvantages of tracheostomy over translaryngeal intubation
   a. Immediate surgical complications in 20% of patients (pneumothorax, subcutaneous emphysema)
   b. Late complications (including innominate artery hemorrhage and tracheal stenosis)
4. Recommendations for tracheostomy
   Long-term mechanical ventilation (projected to be >2–3 weeks):
   a. To improve patient comfort
   b. To simplify airway care
   c. To decrease risk of inadvertent extubation
   d. To provide capacity for speech and oral nutrition
   e. Neurologic patients (e.g., coma) who cannot perceive comfort have increased tracheal injury. In such cases, the usefulness of tracheostomy is questionable.

D. Airway cuff management
1. Use low-pressure–high-compliance cuffs.
2. Maintain cuff pressures at 15–20 mm Hg.
3. Obtain frequent chest radiographs. (Cuff to trachea ratio of >1.5:1 may suggest overdistention).

Figure 22

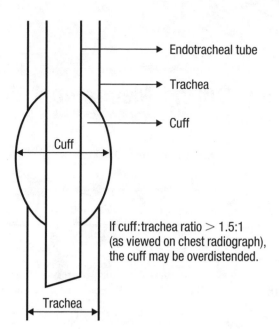

Endotracheal tube

Trachea

Cuff

Cuff

Trachea

If cuff:trachea ratio > 1.5:1
(as viewed on chest radiograph),
the cuff may be overdistended.

12. Monitoring During Mechanical Ventilation

Suhail Raoof, MD

- **Lung mechanics**
- **Peak and plateau pressures**
- **Effective dynamic and static compliance**
- **Clinical applications of compliance measurements**
- **Auto-PEEP**
- **Influence of PEEP on wedge pressures**

A. Lung mechanics

By looking at two pressures on the ventilator dial or digital display, one may obtain valuable information regarding the state of the airways and the lung parenchyma. For this purpose, let us consider an intubated patient connected to a ventilator. Let us imagine that the system (patient and ventilator) is composed of two units:

1. Conducting unit
   a. Includes ventilator tubing, ET-tube, and patient's airways
   b. Is responsible for the resistive properties
2. Lung parenchyma
   a. Contributes to the elastic properties of the respiratory system

Figure 23

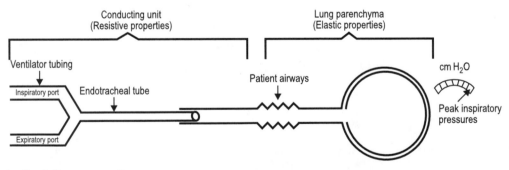

3. Peak Inspiratory Pressures
   When a VT is delivered to the patient, there is a rapid increase in airway pressures. When pressure reaches a maximum at the end of inspiration, it is called *peak inspiratory pressure* (PIP). The PIP reflects the airways resistance and elasticity of the respiratory system. Thus, the greater the airways resistance, or the stiffer the lungs, the higher the PIP.

Figure 24

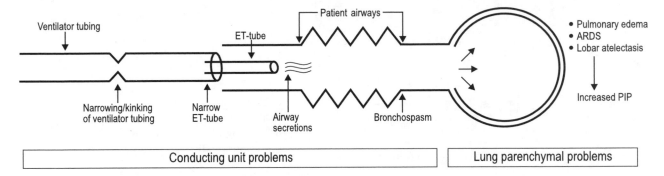

Conducting unit problems | Lung parenchymal problems

When the PIP is high, how can we distinguish whether the problem is in the airways or in the lung parenchyma?

4. Plateau pressures or end-inspiratory static pressures

At the end of inspiration (when the entire VT has been delivered), a newer lower pressure is recorded in the system if the expiratory port is occluded. This is the plateau pressure. To obtain plateau pressure, an end-inspiratory pause of ≥1.0 second is set for one breath. Patient must be passively ventilated for accurate estimation. In this occluded state, no flow is occurring. Because airways resistance is flow dependent, in a no-flow state airways resistance becomes negligible. Thus, the plateau pressures are a reflection of the compliance (or stiffness) of the respiratory system (lung parenchyma and chest wall). The stiffer the lungs, the higher the plateau pressures recorded.

Figure 25

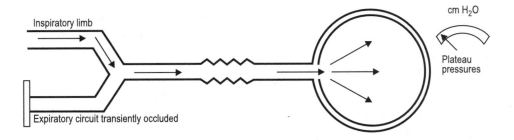

Figure 26

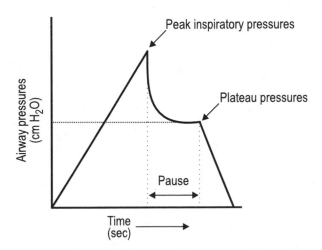

Interpretation of Peak and Plateau Pressure

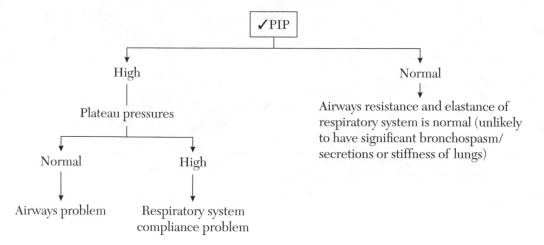

5. Compliance
   a. Volume change per unit pressure change is called *compliance*.
   b. Two compliance measurements are important for a mechanically ventilated patient:

   i. Effective dynamic compliance (Cdyn) $= \dfrac{\text{Change in volume}}{\text{Change in PIP}}$

   where
      change in volume = V_T
   and
      change in PIPs = PIP − baseline pressures.
   Baseline pressure = 0 for most patients or PEEP (intrinsic or extrinsic)
   Thus

   $$Cdyn = \frac{V_T}{PIP - PEEP}$$

   Cdyn is low whenever a patient has an airways or a lung parenchymal problem.

   ii. Static compliance $= \dfrac{\text{Change in volume}}{\text{Change in Pel from baseline}}$

   where
      change in volume = V_T
   and
      change in Pel = Pel − baseline pressure.
   Baseline pressure = 0 or PEEP
   Thus

   $$Cst = \frac{V_T}{Pel - PEEP}$$

   Cst will be normal in patients with airways problems, but low in patients with a lung parenchymal problem.
   c. Normal values of compliance of respiratory system.

   $$Cst = 70\text{--}100 \text{ mL/cm } H_2O$$

   and

   $$Cdyn = 40\text{--}70 \text{ mL/cm } H_2O$$

d. Clinical problem:

A patient who has had an overdose of heroin is brought to the MICU and intubated.

Ventilator settings: CMV—RR of 14 breaths/min/VT 800 mL

Peak pressures: PIP = 20 cm H_2O

Plateau pressures: Pel = 10 cm H_2O

Thus

$$Cdyn = VT/PIP - PEEP = \frac{800 \text{ mL}}{20 - 0 \text{ cm } H_2O}$$

$$= \boxed{40 \text{ mL/cm } H_2O}$$

and

$$Cst = VT/Plateau - PEEP = \frac{800 \text{ mL}}{10 - 0 \text{ cm } H_2O}$$

$$= \boxed{80 \text{ mL/cm } H_2O}$$

Inference: Cst = normal; Cdyn = normal.

If patient's condition deteriorates, ventilator alarms start sounding; record PIP and Pels. New pressures are:

Example 1	Example 2
If: PIP = 40 cm H_2O Pel = 10 cm H_2O ↓ Cst = 800/10 − 0 = 80 mL/cm H_2O (normal) Cdyn = 800/40 − 0 = 20 mL/cm H_2O (low) *Then*: Problem is most likely in the airways (e.g., secretions, bronchospasm)	*If*: PIP = 40 cm H_2O Pel = 35 cm H_2O ↓ Cst = 800/35 − 0 = 22.9 mL/cm H_2O (low) Cdyn = 800/40 − 0 = 20 mL/cm H_2O (low) *Then*: Problem is most likely in the lung parenchyma (e.g., pulmonary edema, ARDS)

Thus, if both the PIP and Pel rise from the baseline, the problem is likely to be in the lung parenchyma. If the PIP increases and the Pel remains normal, the problem is likely to be in the airways.

6. Applications of compliance measurements
   a. Airways versus lung parenchymal problems

Figure 27

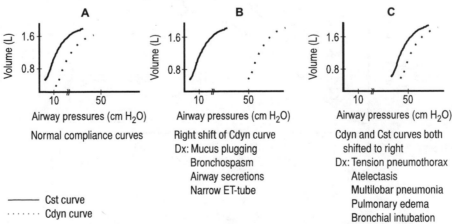

Diagnosis of Causes for Acute Respiratory Distress by Using Pressure Volume Curves

(Modified with permission from Bone RC. Monitoring patients in acute respiratory failure. Respir Care. 1983;28:600.)

b. Calculation of airways resistance
    i. PIP reflects both the airways resistance and the state of respiratory system compliance.
    ii. Pel reflects the state of respiratory system compliance.
    iii. Thus, PIP − Pel reflects the airways resistance.
        So, airways resistance may be estimated by:

$$\frac{\text{PIP} - \text{Pel}}{\text{Peak inspiratory flow (L/sec)}}$$

        This is a useful measure in patients with bronchospasm
c. Weaning index
    i. The stiffer the lungs—i.e., the lower their compliance—the more work of breathing the patient will have to do to inflate lungs during inspiration.
    ii. Hence, a static compliance of the respiratory system of ≤25 mL/cm H_2O is a poor weaning index.
d. Predicting barotrauma
    i. PIP
        a) PIP is a poor indicator of volutrauma. High peak inspiratory pressures dissipate in the larger airways.
        b) Very high PIPs may, however, be transmitted to the alveoli.
    ii. Pel
        a) Pel is the best estimate of maximum alveolar pressures.
        b) Pel >35 cm H_2O may predict development of volutrauma (especially in patients with intrinsic lung disease).
e. Calculating optimal PEEP
    i. One of the definitions of optimal PEEP is the lowest level of PEEP that results in the maximum recruitment of alveoli without overdistention.
    ii. At the point of optimal alveolar recruitment, the lungs should be maximally compliant.
    iii. To calculate optimal PEEP using this technique, add PEEP in small increments and calculate the Cst.
    iv. The level or range of PEEP that results in the highest static compliance is likely to be the optimal PEEP.

Figure 28

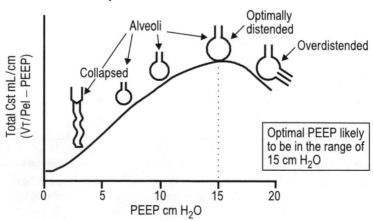

Optimal PEEP Determination

f. Calculating pressure support
   i. Pressure support is sometimes given to overcome the resistance of the ventilator circuit and the endotracheal tube.
   ii. In such situations, requisite level of pressure support may be calculated by:

$$\frac{PIP - Pel}{Peak\ inspiratory\ flow}$$

For example, if

$$PIP = 30\ cm\ H_2O$$

and

$$Pel = 20\ cm\ H_2O$$

and

$$Peak\ inspiratory\ flows = 60\ L/min = 1\ L/sec$$

then appropriate pressure support may be $30 - 20\ cm\ H_2O = 10\ cm\ of\ H_2O$

B. Auto-PEEP (occult or intrinsic PEEP)
1. Concept
   a. In the presence of increased airway resistance, a high demand for ventilation, or a short expiratory time, air flow may still occur at end exhalation. Thus, pressure in the alveoli is still positive at end exhalation—i.e., auto-PEEP.
   b. Auto-PEEP should be suspected if the flow tracings on the ventilator reveal continuous expiratory flow until the start of inspiratory flow.
2. Definitions
   a. Dynamic hyperinflation: a phenomenon in which the lung volume measured just before the initiation of inspiration is greater than the passive FRC.

Figure 29

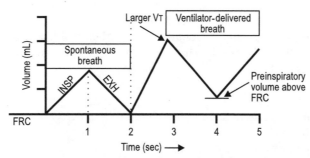

   b. Auto-PEEP: the difference between the mean alveolar pressure and external airway pressure at end exhalation measured when the patient is not making any respiratory excursions (passive ventilation)

Figure 30

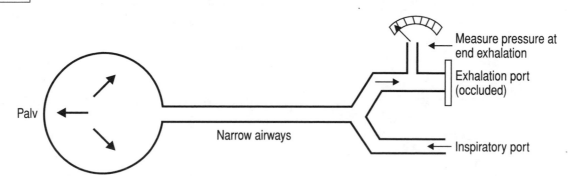

3. Causes of auto-PEEP
    a. Expiratory flow limitation
        i. Intrinsic pulmonary problem (e.g., COPD/acute asthma)
        ii. Nonpulmonary problem (e.g., narrow endotracheal tube, long ventilator tubing)
    b. Increased flow resistance (e.g., ARDS)
    c. High $\dot{V}E$ (>12–15 L/min)
        i. Patient driven (e.g., trauma, stroke, severe metabolic acidosis)
        ii. Ventilator driven (increased rate or V_T)
4. Practical example of auto-PEEP
    A patient with exacerbation of COPD is intubated and mechanically ventilated. Ventilator settings include:
    Assist/control mode (volume targeted)
        V_T = 1000 mL
        RR (no spontaneous patient breaths) = 20 breaths/min
        Inspiratory flow rate = 1000 mL/sec (or 60 L/min)
        Thus, time for 1 breath (inspiration + exhalation) = 60 sec/20 breaths = 3 sec/breath
        Because flow rate = 1000 mL/sec, it will take 1 second to deliver the V_T volume of 1000 mL.
        Thus, time for inspiration = 1 second; time for exhalation = 3 − 1 = 2 seconds.
        If the patient has bronchospasm, 2 seconds for exhalation may not allow the entire 1000 mL V_T to come out of the lungs.
        Let us suppose that only 500 mL of air has come out at the end of 2 seconds of exhalation. Hence, at the end of exhalation:
        • Flow will still be occurring
        • Lung volume will be greater than expected (compared with the normal equilibrium state of FRC).
        • Pressure will still be positive in the alveoli.
        At the end of 3 seconds (1 second for inspiration and 2 seconds for exhalation), the ventilator will deliver another V_T of 1000 mL.
        So at the end of the second V_T delivery, the patient will have 500 mL of air (remaining from first breath) + 1000 mL. This will result in progressive dynamic hyperinflation.
5. Values of intrinsic PEEP clinically encountered*
    a. Patients with COPD
        i. Stable
            a) Spontaneously breathing: usually up to 9 cm H_2O
        ii. Exacerbation
            a) Spontaneously breathing: usually up to 13 cm H_2O
            b) Mechanically ventilated: usually up to 22 cm H_2O
    b. Asthma patients
        i. Exacerbation
            a) Mechanically ventilated: usually up to 22 cm H_2O
    c. Pulmonary edema
        i. Mechanically ventilated: usually up to 8 cm H_2O

* Data from Milic-Emili J. How to monitor PEEP and why. J Crit Care Illness. 1992;7:25-32.

Figure 31

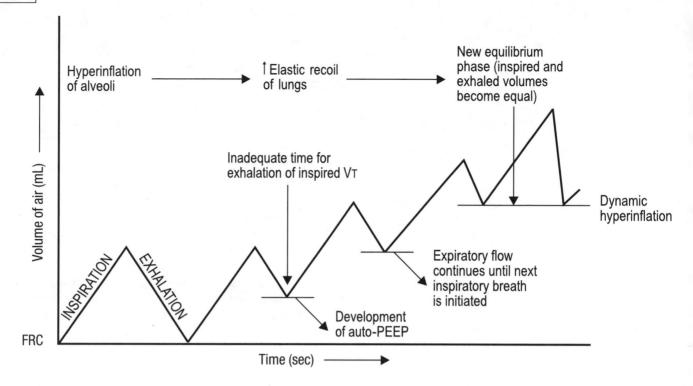

6. Method of measuring auto-PEEP
   (Unlike ventilator PEEP, auto-PEEP does not reflect on the ventilator pressure manometer)
   a. On the ventilator
      i. End exhalation occlusion technique

Figure 32

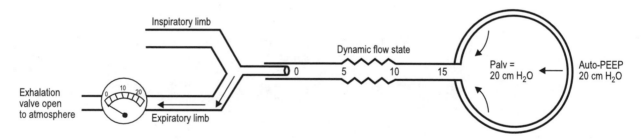

Airways resistance is flow dependent.

As a result of the airways resistance, the alveolar pressure at end exhalation (20 cm H_2O) is dissipated in the central airways.

Thus, airway pressures measured at the exhalation port may be negligible (0 in this case).

Figure 33

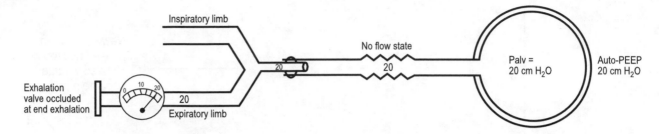

When the exhalation valve is occluded (at end exhalation), a no-flow state is created.
Because airways resistance is flow dependent, in a no-flow state, airways resistance becomes negligible.
Thus, no dissipation of pressures occurs in the central airways.
So, the alveolar pressure (Palv) equilibrates in the airways and is accurately reflected by the manometer at the exhalation port.
This positive pressure at end exhalation reflects the auto-PEEP.

    ii. Measure Pel for one isolated breath during volume-targeted ventilation (at usual set rate). Put patient on CPAP for 30 seconds, then switch to volume-targeted ventilation and measure Pel again for the first few breaths. The difference in readings between the two Pels is a rough indication of auto-PEEP.

    iii. When inspiration is triggered by ventilator: the pressure generated by the ventilator to initiate inspiratory flow reflects the auto-PEEP.

  b. Spontaneous breathing

    i. Negative esophageal pressure developed just before the beginning of inspiratory flow is an indicator of auto-PEEP.

7. Effects of auto-PEEP

  a.

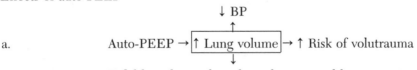

Tidal breathing takes place close to total lung capacity where respiratory compliance is low

  b. Increased work of breathing

Figure 34

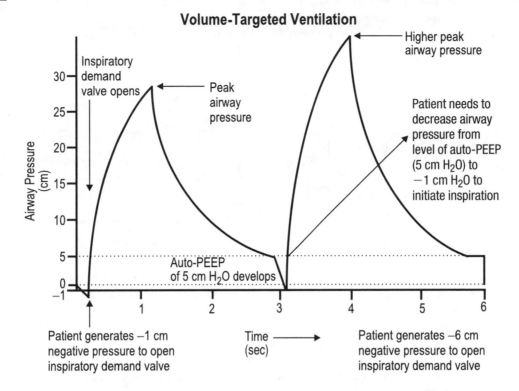

Volume-Targeted Ventilation

Inspiratory demand valve opens

Peak airway pressure

Higher peak airway pressure

Patient needs to decrease airway pressure from level of auto-PEEP (5 cm H$_2$O) to −1 cm H$_2$O to initiate inspiration

Auto-PEEP of 5 cm H$_2$O develops

Airway Pressure (cm)

Time (sec)

Patient generates −1 cm negative pressure to open inspiratory demand valve

Patient generates −6 cm negative pressure to open inspiratory demand valve

    i. The patient needs to generate enough negative pressure to offset the auto-PEEP and reach the inspiratory trigger threshold. This may cause:
      a) Inspiratory muscle fatigue
      b) Failure to wean
c. Decreased efficiency of generation of force by respiratory muscles.

Laplace Law states:

$$\text{Pressure} = \frac{2 \times \text{Tension}}{\text{Radius of curvature}} = \frac{2T}{r}$$

Auto-PEEP → hyperinflation → flattening of diaphragms

Figure 35

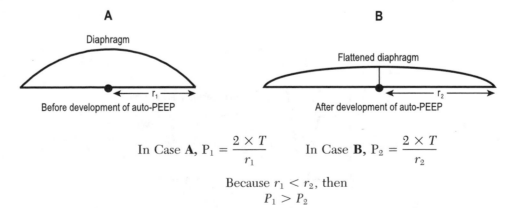

A

Diaphragm

r_1

Before development of auto-PEEP

B

Flattened diaphragm

r_2

After development of auto-PEEP

In Case **A**, $P_1 = \dfrac{2 \times T}{r_1}$ In Case **B**, $P_2 = \dfrac{2 \times T}{r_2}$

Because $r_1 < r_2$, then
$$P_1 > P_2$$

(i.e., the pressure generated by the diaphragm retaining its normal radius of curvature is expected to be greater than the pressure it can generate when flattened, as in hyperinflation states).

    d. Erroneous measurements of:
       i. Pulmonary capillary wedge pressure
       ii. Respiratory system compliance
    e. Decreased VT delivery in pressure-targeted ventilation (see Fig. 36)

Figure 36

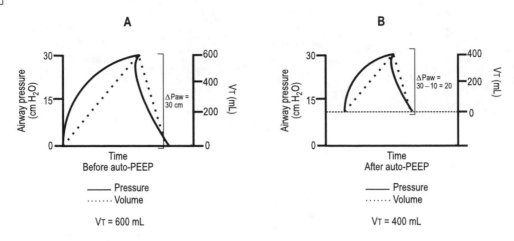

A

B

VT = 600 mL

VT = 400 mL

    f. Hypercapnic respiratory failure*
    $Paco_2$ (mm Hg) $= 36.8 + 1.56 \times$ intrinsic PEEP (cm H_2O)
    (Thus, 1 cm of intrinsic PEEP may result in a 1.56 mm Hg increase in $Paco_2$)
    *Data from Milic-Emili J. How to monitor intrinsic PEEP and why. J Crit Care Illness. 1992;7:25-32.
8. Strategies for minimizing auto-PEEP
    a. Relieve obstruction (inhaled bronchodilators)
    b. Sedate ± paralyze
    c. Decrease $\dot{V}E$ (rate and VT)
    d. Increase peak inspiratory flow rate
    e. Resort to permissive hypercapnia
    f. Use PEEP (slightly less than auto-PEEP)
       i. May keep airways patent
       ii. Decreases inspiratory work of breathing. Consider the example in Fig. 37 of a patient with auto-PEEP (10 cm H_2O) and no extrinsic or set PEEP. This patient must generate a negative inspiratory pressure of −11 cm H_2O to initiate inspiration from the ventilator.

Figure 37

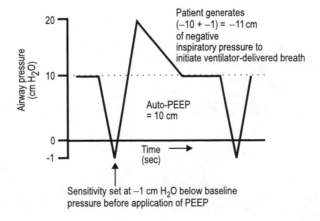

    In Figure 38, an extrinsic PEEP of 8 cm H_2O is set. In order to generate −1 cm H_2O

pressure below the baseline of 8 cm H_2O, the patient must bring the airway pressure to 7 cm H_2O. Thus, to lower the airway pressure from 10 cm H_2O to 7 cm H_2O, the patient must generate -3 cm H_2O negative inspiratory pressure. Application of PEEP slightly less than intrinsic PEEP has thereby resulted in significant reduction in work of breathing.

Figure 38

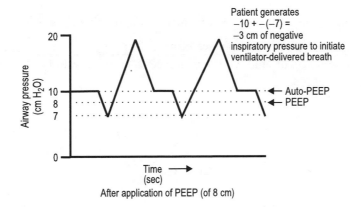

Patient generates
$-10 + -(-7) =$
-3 cm of negative
inspiratory pressure to initiate
ventilator-delivered breath

Auto-PEEP
PEEP

Airway pressure (cm H_2O)

Time (sec)
After application of PEEP (of 8 cm)

9. Practical tips
  a. Auto-PEEP is not uniform in all lung units. It is greater in lung units with higher airways resistance (those that empty slowly). Thus, auto-PEEP of a particular level is not the same as PEEP of a similar level.
  b. Auto-PEEP depicts the average end-exhalation airways pressure.
C. Influence of PEEP on pulmonary artery occlusion pressure (PAOP) or wedge pressure
  True PAOP = observed PAOP (wedge pressure) from right-heart catheter − juxtacardiac pressure
  Juxtacardiac pressure = pressure exerted on the heart by the lungs.

Figure 39

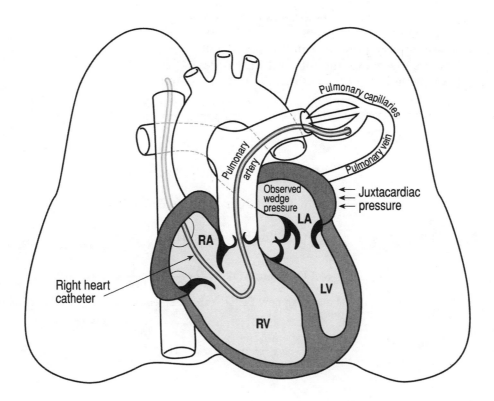

Pulmonary capillaries
Pulmonary vein
Pulmonary artery
Observed wedge pressure
Juxtacardiac pressure
LA
RA
Right heart catheter
LV
RV

The greater the degree of lung inflation, the greater is the juxtacardiac pressure, and hence the greater is the observed PAOP (wedge pressure).

To minimize the influence of juxtacardiac pressures on the PAOP, the PAOP is measured at end exhalation.

With the least inflation of lungs at end exhalation, the effects of alveolar distention on wedge pressure will be minimized.

However, juxtacardiac pressure at end exhalation may still be significant if the patient has intrinsic or extrinsic PEEP.

Juxtacardiac pressure will then be estimated by mean pleural pressure ($\overline{\text{Ppl}}$):

$$\overline{\text{Ppl}} = \frac{\text{Compliance of lung (CL)}}{\text{Compliance of lung (CL)} + \text{Compliance of chest wall (Cw)}} \times \text{PEEP}$$

So,

$$\overline{\text{Ppl}} = \frac{\text{CL}}{\text{CL} + \text{Cw}}$$

Normally,

$$\text{CL} = \text{Cw}$$

So,

$$\overline{\text{Ppl}} = \frac{\text{CL}}{\text{CL} + \text{CL}} \times \text{PEEP} = \frac{\text{CL}}{2\,\text{CL}} \times \text{PEEP} = \frac{1}{2}\,\text{PEEP}$$

Thus, pleural pressure transmitted to the heart is estimated by 1/2 PEEP.

For example,

if

$$\text{PEEP} = 10 \text{ cm H}_2\text{O}$$

and

$$\text{PAOP} = 20 \text{ mm Hg} = 27 \text{ cm H}_2\text{O} \ (1 \text{ mm Hg} = 1.36 \text{ cm H}_2\text{O})$$

then

$$\text{true PAOP will be } 27 \text{ cm H}_2\text{O} - 1/2 \times 10 = 22 \text{ cm H}_2\text{O} = 16.2 \text{ mm Hg}$$

Other formulae used to get estimations of true PAOP are:
a. In ARDS, true PAOP = observed PAOP $- 0.5 \times$ (PEEP $- 10$)
b. Measure wedge pressure with PEEP = PAOP_1
   Measure wedge pressure without PEEP = PAOP_2
   Decrease in PAOP (due to PEEP) = $\text{PAOP}_1 - \text{PAOP}_2$

$$\text{Expressed as percentage of PEEP} = \frac{\text{PAOP}_1 - \text{PAOP}_2}{\text{PEEP}}$$

For example,
if

$$\text{PAOP}_1 = 15 \text{ mm Hg} = 20 \text{ cm H}_2\text{O}$$

and

$$\text{PAOP}_2 = 12 \text{ mm Hg} = 16 \text{ cm H}_2\text{O}$$

and

$$\text{PEEP} = 12 \text{ cm H}_2\text{O}$$

Then,

$$\text{the influence of PEEP on PAOP} = \frac{20 - 16}{12} = \frac{4}{12} = 33\% \text{ of PEEP}$$

If this patient were to be given a new PEEP level of 20 cm H$_2$O, the PAOP may increase by

$$\frac{20 \times 33}{100} = 6.6 \text{ cm H}_2\text{O}$$

13. Weaning from Mechanical Ventilation

Suhail Raoof, MD

- Definition
- Broad criteria and guidelines
- Factors that should be corrected
- Methods of weaning
- Guidelines for weaning
- Extubation protocol guidelines
- Difficult-to-wean patients (algorithm)

A. **Definition**

Switching from mechanical to spontaneous ventilation.

B. **Broad criteria**
1. Reversal of initial process that led to respiratory failure
2. Correction of nonpulmonary factors
3. Assessment of adequacy of ventilatory parameters

C. **Guidelines**
1. After short ventilatory support (3–7 days)
   a. No underlying lung disease
   b. No nutritional deficiencies
   c. No major organ failure
   Quick wean: T-piece trial can be attempted.
2. After long-term ventilatory support (>1 week). Reasons that commonly preclude weaning include:
   a. Underlying lung disease
   b. Nutritional deficiencies
   c. Major organ failure
Quick weaning may be attempted. Some patients may require slower weaning using SIMV, PSV, or daily T-piece trials.

D. **Factors that should be corrected *before* weaning, if possible.**
1. Nonpulmonary
   a. CNS
      i. Impaired level of consciousness
      ii. Excessive need for sedatives and narcotic analgesics
      iii. Absence of gag reflex
      iv. Absence of cough reflex
      v. Sleep deprivation
   b. CVS
      i. Shock
      ii. Arrhythmias
   c. Renal/electrolytes
      i. Volume overload (SIADH)
      ii. Metabolic alkalosis (results in alveolar hypoventilation on extubation with atelectasis, leftward shift of oxygen dissociation curve)

iii. Posthypercapnic metabolic alkalosis in patients with CO_2 retention

iv. Metabolic acidosis (increased $\dot{V}E$)

d. Hematologic

i. Anemia (decreased oxygen-carrying capacity)

e. Infections

i. High fevers/infection (increased CO_2 production requiring higher $\dot{V}E$)

f. Nutrition

i. Poor nutritional status

ii. Low phosphorus (less than 1 mg/dL) − [muscular weakness, diaphragmatic atrophy, depressed respiratory drive, increased susceptibility to infections]

iii. Excessive nutrition

iv. High carbohydrate load [increased $\dot{V}E$ requirements]

2. Pulmonary (weaning parameters)

Component Assessed and Rationale	Weaning Index	Description	Weaning Outcome		Predicted Value	
			Good	Poor	PPV	NPV
1. **Respiratory muscle pump** • **Respiratory muscle strength** Commonest cause of failure to wean May be caused by inspiratory muscle weakness or neuromuscular disorders	**Commonly used** *i*) Maximum inspiratory pressure (PImax)	PImax generated by a patient from FRC approximately 20 sec after occluding the inspiratory circuit. May be performed in non-cooperative patients.	More negative than −30 cm H_2O	Less negative than −20 cm H_2O	0.58–0.71	0.55–1.0
	ii) Index of rapid shallow breathing RR/VT	Inspiratory muscle weakness leads to rapid shallow breathing. The patient is disconnected from the ventilator for 1 minute. The respiratory rate (breaths/min) is divided by the spontaneous VT (in liters). Measurements are usually made by a bedside spirometer.	<100 breaths/ min/L	>100 breaths/ min/L	0.78	0.95
	iii) Paradoxic breathing	Normally both the chest and the abdomen move outward when the patient inspires. Paradoxic movement of the *thorax* indicates intercostal muscle fatigue; paradoxic movement of the *abdomen,* diaphragmatic fatigue.	Absence of paradoxic thoracic and abdominal wall movement	Presence of paradoxic thoracic and abdominal wall movement	—	—

(continues)

Component Assessed and Rationale	Weaning Index	Description	Weaning Outcome		Predicted Value	
			Good	Poor	PPV	NPV
• **Respiratory muscle strength—cont'd**	*iv*) Respiratory alterans	A paradoxic movement of the abdomen that alternates with paradoxic movement of the thorax on a breath by breath basis. Indicates diaphragmatic fatigue.	Absent	Present	1.0	0.96
	Less commonly used					
	v) Vital capacity (VC)	The maximum amount of a gas that can be inhaled from residual volume or exhaled from total lung capacity. VC is an integrative index that requires patient comprehension, respiratory muscle output, and the state of compliance and resistance of the respiratory system. Normal VC = 65–75 mL/kg of body weight. It cannot predict if the respiratory muscles will be able to carry out the work of breathing over a period of time. However, the closer the spontaneous V_T is to the vital capacity ($V_T/VC > 0.4$), the greater the likelihood of fatigue. Greatest disadvantage is that performing the maneuver requires the cooperation of the patient.	VC >15 mL/kg body weight or V_T/VC <0.4	VC <10 mL/kg body weight or V_T/VC >0.4	Same as PImax	Same as PImax

(continues)

Component Assessed and Rationale	Weaning Index	Description	Weaning Outcome		Predicted Value	
			Good	Poor	PPV	NPV
• **Respiratory muscle strength—**cont'd	*vi*) Diaphragmatic electromyogram	The electromyographic power spectrum indicates the frequency characteristics of complex waves. For the diaphragm, most of the power spectrum is between 20 and 250 Hz. Under normal circumstances, there is a fixed ratio between high and low frequencies. A decrease in high-to-low frequency ratio indicates diaphragmatic fatigue—i.e., the power spectrum shifts from 125–250 Hz to low frequencies (20–50 Hz). By using EMG recordings, the ventilator settings that allow suppression of spontaneous diaphragmatic activity may allow complete rest of the diaphragm.	No shift in power spectrum on surface recordings	Power spectral shift on surface recordings	—	—
	vii) Airway occlusion pressure (P 0.1)	The airway pressure measured 0.1 sec after initiating inspiration against an occluded airway is a reflection of the respiratory drive. The value may be obtained in both unconscious and conscious patients. Although the P 0.1 is an index of respiratory drive, increased values reflect respiratory distress. Thus, an increased P 0.1 value mirrors the response of the respiratory center to deteriorating lung function. In normal individuals, P 0.1 value is <2 cm H_2O.	<2 cm H_2O or doubling of P 0.1 values from breathing at rest to breathing 3% CO_2	>4.2 cm H_2O	—	—

(continues)

Component Assessed and Rationale	Weaning Index	Description	Weaning Outcome		Predicted Value	
			Good	Poor	PPV	NPV
• **Respiratory muscle demands** Respiratory muscle strength may be adequate at a point in time; however, if the work load on the respiratory muscles is increased, they may fatigue over a period of time. The amount of work performed by the respiratory muscles is a function of: *a*) airways resistance *b*) respiratory system compliance *c*) minute volume	**Commonly used** *i*) Static (respiratory system) Compliance (Cst)	Work must be performed by the inspiratory muscles to overcome the elastic properties of both the lungs and chest wall. The stiffer the lungs are, or the more deformed the chest wall is, the more the work of breathing. An assessment of the work of breathing can be made by looking at the thoracic static compliance (Cst) = $$\frac{\text{Tidal volume (V\textsc{t})}}{\text{Plateau pressure (Pel)} - \text{PEEP}}$$ Its major advantage is that it is not effort dependent.	>33 mL/cm H_2O	<25 mL/cm H_2O	0.60	0.53
	ii) Minute ventilation ($\dot{V}_E$)	The amount of air that must be moved in or out of the lungs over 1 minute to maintain a given $Paco_2$ (40 mm Hg). Its major disadvantage is that it is highly effort dependent. Now $$Paco_2 = \frac{\dot{V}co_2}{\dot{V}_A} \times K$$ or $$\dot{V}_E = \frac{Vco_2}{Paco_2\,(1 - V_D/V_T)}$$ (see section on commonly used formulae). Hence, to maintain a constant $Paco_2$, the $\dot{V}_E$ will be determined by the CO_2 production and the V_D/V_T. If CO_2 production is increased (critical illness, high fever, overfeeding or excess carbohydrate load) or V_D/V_T is increased (as in $\dot{V}/\dot{Q}$ mismatch of COPD, ARDS, etc.), the patient will need to do more work of breathing. Thus, the patient is less likely to keep up the spontaneous work of breathing for a period of time.	<10 L/min	>10 L/min	0.50	0.40

(continues)

Component Assessed and Rationale	Weaning Index	Description	Weaning Outcome		Predicted Value	
			Good	**Poor**	**PPV**	**NPV**
• **Respiratory muscle demands— cont'd**	*iii*) Respiratory rate (RR)	As the inspiratory muscles fatigue, the patient resorts to rapid and shallow breathing. In a study by Tobin and colleagues (1986) it was determined that all patients who failed weaning trials had an RR >25 breaths/min.	≤35 breaths/min	>35 breaths/min	0.65 (for RR ≥38 breaths/min)	0.77 (for RR ≤38 breaths/min)
	Less commonly used					
	iv) Maximum voluntary ventilation (MVV)	The maximum amount of air that can be inhaled or exhaled over 1 minute is the MVV. The relationship between $\dot{V}_E$ and MVV provides a weaning index. If a person is able to double the $\dot{V}_E$ during an MVV measurement, it indicates that the patient has adequate respiratory reserve. The major disadvantage is that the test requires a cooperative and motivated patient who can coordinate the maneuver.	MVV > two times the $\dot{V}_E$	MVV < two times the $\dot{V}_E$	0.95	0.24
	v) Dead space ventilation (V_D/V_T)	The ratio of V_D/V_T is a reflection of wasted ventilation. Because $V_T = V_A + V_D$ or $V_A = V_T - V_D$, the greater the V_D, the greater should be the V_T to maintain a constant V_A. Normally, the V_D/V_T is between 0.33 and 0.45. A number of clinical conditions like COPD and ARDS increase the V_D/V_T and hence the work of breathing.	<0.6	≥0.6	—	—

(continues)

Component Assessed and Rationale	Weaning Index	Description	Weaning Outcome		Predicted Value	
			Good	Poor	PPV	NPV
• **Respiratory muscle demands—cont'd**	*vi*) CO_2 production ($\dot{V}CO_2$)	Because $$PaCO_2 = \frac{\dot{V}CO_2}{\dot{V}E\,(1 - VD/VT)}$$ if $\dot{V}CO_2$ increases, the $\dot{V}E$ will need to increase to prevent the $PaCO_2$ from rising. A hypermetabolic state (such as fever, thyrotoxicosis, sepsis, seizures) will increase the ventilatory demands, and it may culminate in respiratory muscle fatigue. The mixed expired CO_2 fraction of the exhaled gases in 1 min indicates the $\dot{V}CO_2$.	<200 mL/min	>250 mL/min	—	—
	vii) Work of breathing (WOB)	It is important to determine the level of respiratory work that a patient needs to perform to sustain spontaneous breathing. In certain other situations, where the patient may be failing the weaning trial, it may be useful to assess the (unmeasured) work of breathing imposed by the breathing circuit (ET-tube, ventilator tubing, ventilator demand valve). WOB has been considered by some as the best weaning index. It takes into consideration the pressure work to overcome the airways resistance, elastic properties of the respiratory system, and the minute ventilation.	—	—	—	—

(continues)

Component Assessed and Rationale	Weaning Index	Description	Weaning Outcome		Predicted Value	
			Good	Poor	PPV	NPV
• Respiratory muscle demands—cont'd	General indicators of WOB					
	• Airways resistance = $\dfrac{PIP - Pel}{PIF\ (L/sec)}$	See section on Airways Resistance in Monitoring During Mechanical Ventilation on (p 60).	<5 cm H_2O/L/sec	>5 cm H_2O/L/sec	—	—
	• Negative deflection of airway pressure gauge of the ventilator	Significant negative deflection of the airway pressure gauge from the baseline (end exhalation) value may be indicative of increased inspiratory work of breathing. Common causes include decreased sensitivity of inspiratory demand valve, low flow rates, and long inspiratory time delay. This negative deflection of the pressure gauge in conjunction with tachypnea, diaphoresis, or the use of inspiratory accessory muscles may indicate the development of muscle fatigue in a person being weaned.	—	—	—	—
	Specific indicators of WOB					
	• O_2 cost of breathing (expressed as percentage of total work of breathing)	The difference between the O_2 consumption of a spontaneously breathing patient and the O_2 cost of breathing in a patient receiving mechanical ventilation. The greater the O_2 cost of breathing, the less is the likelihood of weaning success. These measurements can be made using a microprocessor-based monitor and esophageal balloon.	<9% of total body O_2 consumption	>39% of total body O_2 consumption	1.0	0.63

(continues)

2. Pulmonary (weaning parameters)—cont'd

Component Assessed and Rationale	Weaning Index	Description	Weaning Outcome		Predicted Value	
			Good	Poor	PPV	NPV
• Respiratory muscle demands—cont'd	• O_2 cost of breathing (expressed as work/min or kg × m/min)	Same as above	<1.34 kg × m/min	>1.34 kg × m/min	0.84	0.84
	• O_2 cost of breathing (expressed as work/L or kg × m/L)	Same as above	<0.10 kg × m/L	≥0.10 kg × m/L	Same as above	Same as above
2. **Respiratory gas exchange*** Significant hypoxemia constitutes a relative contraindication to weaning. The weaning phase may be associated with smaller tidal volumes, atelectasis, and worsening hypoxemia. A PaO_2 <60 mm Hg with an FIO_2 >0.40 is usually considered a relative contraindication to weaning.	*i*) Arterial to inspired O_2 ratio (PaO_2/FIO_2)	The partial pressure of O_2 in the arterial blood is a direct reflection of the fraction of O_2 in the inspired gases. However, if there is a $\dot{V}/\dot{Q}$ mismatch, diffusion abnormality, or shunt, hypoxemia may set in. PaO_2/FIO_2 ratio is easily calculated, but its major disadvantage is it does not take into account the influence of $PaCO_2$ on PaO_2.	>200	<200	0.90	0.10
	ii) Arterial to alveolar O_2 tension (PaO_2/PAO_2)	The value of PAO_2 can be calculated from the alveolar gas equation: $$PAO_2 = PIO_2 - \frac{PaCO_2}{R}$$ Its advantages are that it changes less with varying FIO_2 and can be derived from arterial blood gases. It may be affected by determinants of $P\bar{v}O_2$, Hb, $\dot{V}O_2$, $\dot{D}O_2$.	>0.35	<0.35	0.59	0.53
	iii) Alveolar arterial oxygen gradient [(A − a) O_2]	Normally, O_2 diffuses passively down its concentration gradient from the alveoli to the pulmonary capillaries. Conditions causing gas exchange problems at the alveolar level (i.e., excluding hypoventilation and pure hypercapnic respiratory failure) may result in significant increase in (A − a)O_2.	<350 mm Hg	>350 mm Hg	—	—

* Another oxygenation index (OI) = $\dfrac{\overline{Paw} \times FIO_2 \times 100}{PaO_2}$ has been described frequently in neonatal literature. It takes into consideration the mean airway pressure required for a particular level of oxygenation. It has been reported as an indicator of mortality in ARDS (OI >42 at 24 h predicts mortality with a sensitivity of 62% and specificity of 93%—Arnold et al, 1993). However, it has not been studied extensively as a weaning index.

(continues)

Component Assessed and Rationale	Weaning Index	Description	Weaning Outcome		Predicted Value	
			Good	Poor	PPV	NPV
• **Respiratory muscle demands—cont'd**	*iv*) Shunt fraction ($\dot{Q}s/\dot{Q}t$)	Blood that enters the arterial system without going through the ventilated areas of the lung constitutes a shunt: $$\dot{Q}s/\dot{Q}t = \frac{Cc'o_2 - Cao_2}{Cc'o_2 - C\bar{v}o_2}$$ where $Cc'o_2 = O_2$ content of end capillary blood, $Cao_2 = O_2$ content of arterial blood, and $C\bar{v}o_2 = O_2$ content of mixed venous blood.	Shunt fraction <20%	Shunt fraction >20%	—	—
3. **Integrative indices** These indices combine assessment of respiratory work load, respiratory muscle strength, gas exchange, etc. Therefore, they are likely to have greater predictive powers.	*i*) CROP Index C = compliance R = rate O = oxygenation P = pressure	CROP = Cdyn × PImax × [Pao_2/PAo_2] rate	≥13 mL/ breath/min	<13 mL/ breath/min	0.71	0.70
	ii) Simplified weaning index	Simplified weaning index is $$fmv\,\frac{PIP - PEEP}{PImax} \times \frac{Paco_2mv}{40}$$ where fmv = ventilator rate, PIP = peak inspiratory pressure, PEEP = positive end-expiratory pressure, PImax = maximum inspiratory pressure, and $Paco_2mv$ = $Paco_2$ on the ventilator. The index is a simplified version of the weaning index (WI). It is less accurate than WI (especially if values are in a range of 9–11/min). However, it can be easily and rapidly calculated.	<9 min	>11 min	0.93	0.95

3. Proposed weaning parameters that can be easily tested at bedside

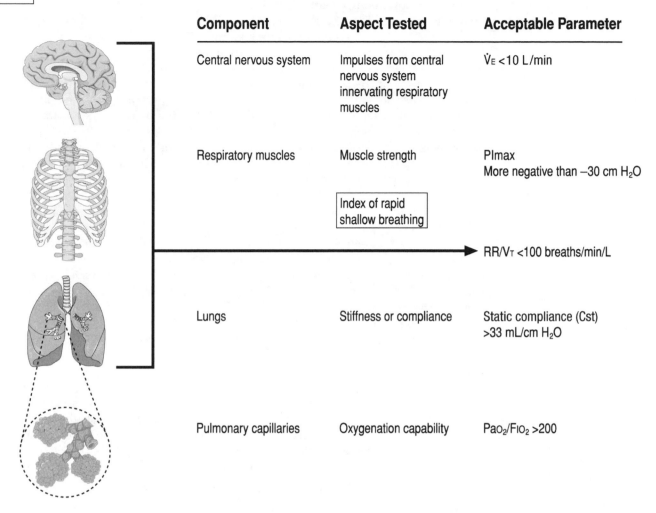

Component	Aspect Tested	Acceptable Parameter
Central nervous system	Impulses from central nervous system innervating respiratory muscles	$\dot{V}_E$ <10 L/min
Respiratory muscles	Muscle strength	PImax More negative than −30 cm H_2O
	Index of rapid shallow breathing	RR/V_T <100 breaths/min/L
Lungs	Stiffness or compliance	Static compliance (Cst) >33 mL/cm H_2O
Pulmonary capillaries	Oxygenation capability	Pa_{O_2}/F_{IO_2} >200

4. Conventionally, studies done by Sahn and others (1976) have shown that the following weaning parameters successfully predicted weaning success:
   a. VC >15 mL/kg
   b. PImax <−20 cm H_2O
   c. $\dot{V}_E$ (for Pa_{CO_2} of 40 mm Hg) <10 L/min
   d. MVV = 2 × $\dot{V}_E$ (i.e., ability to at least double the $\dot{V}_E$)
5. The usefulness of weaning indices varies greatly in the literature. Reasons for variability include:
   a. Differences in the patient populations
   b. Lack of standardization of weaning protocols
   c. Lack of reproducibility of measurements
   d. Different "acceptable values" for weaning parameters
   e. Lack of standardization of end points

E. Methods of weaning
   Considerable variation in techniques of weaning exists. No one method or technique of weaning has been definitely found to be superior. Appropriate time for at least partial reversal of the process that led to institution of mechanical ventilation in the first place should be given. Special consideration should be given to the resistance of the endotracheal tube, airway secretions, work of breathing imposed by the ventilator, and persistence of auto-PEEP. Patients with COPD and chronic ventilatory failure (CO_2 retention) should have gradual reduction in $\dot{V}_E$, if necessary, to allow the Pa_{CO_2} to return to its baseline levels before extubation (see pp 151–153, 155).

Patients with left ventricular failure should have their volume status corrected before weaning is begun (see p 155).

1. **Initial trial of spontaneous breathing**
   a. One way to assess if the patient is ready for rapid weaning is to give a spontaneous breathing trial through a continuous flow circuit providing CPAP or a T-tube for 3–5 minutes and to observe closely the patient's RR and VT.
   b. Some clinicians prefer to overcome the imposed airways resistance of the ET-tube and ventilator circuit by adding an appropriate level of positive pressure with the CPAP mode (usually ≈5 cm H_2O). (An estimation of the airways resistance may be obtained by subtracting the Pel from the PIP and dividing by the peak inspiratory flow rate.)
   c. The advantage of the CPAP technique is that the ventilator circuit does not need to be modified and that the ventilator alarms and apnea ventilation option are available for the patient who stops breathing.
   d. The FIO_2 is usually kept at the pre-trial level.
   e. For the T-tube circuit, the gas flow is kept at more than twice the patient's spontaneous V̇E. The gas should be humidified.
   f. At the end of 3–5 minutes, if the patient's RR is <35/min, the heart rate has not changed by >20% from baseline, the spontaneous VT is >5 mL/kg body weight, SaO_2 >90%, no new potentially serious arrhythmias are observed, and the patient is not greatly agitated, diaphoretic, or anxious, the spontaneous breathing trial is continued (for an additional 30 min to 2–3 hours, depending on physician preferences and the clinical condition of the patient).
   g. If the initial spontaneous breathing trial is terminated on clinical grounds, the patient is put back on the ventilator, preferably on assist/control mode.

2. **Gradual weaning**
   If the patient fails the initial trial of spontaneous breathing on clinical grounds, it may be preferable not to attempt another T-tube trial for approximately 24 hours. A more gradual weaning approach is then followed. A gradual approach has some theoretical advantages. It allows gradual reduction of ventilatory support. A more graded reduction of ventilatory support may allow the fatigued respiratory muscles to take over the work of breathing incrementally without invoking further fatigue or muscle dystrophy. These are, however, theoretical considerations and may bear little relevance clinically. The various options include:
   a. T-tube trials
      i. Once daily trials
         a) Patient's clinical status and weaning parameters are checked to assess feasibility of weaning.
         b) The ventilatory support is abruptly discontinued.
         c) T-tube trial is initiated, usually using the same level of FIO_2 and humidified gas.
         d) The recommended length of the T-tube is approximately 12 inches, added to the expiratory tubing, to disallow for entrainment of air.
         e) The duration of the trial is usually set at 1½–2 hours (range ½ h to several hours).
         f) If the patient's clinical condition, especially RR and VT and hemodynamic stability, is maintained, most clinicians will consider getting an arterial blood gas.
         g) A 2-hour T-tube trial, tolerated well by the patient, usually indicates that the patient can be safely extubated.
         h) If the patient develops respiratory muscle fatigue, assist/control mode of mechanical ventilation is instituted and the patient is rested, usually for 24 hours.
      ii. Multiple, intermittent T-tube trials
         a) T-tube trials are carried out generally for an increasing interval of time (e.g., 5–120 min).
         b) These trials may be repeated every 3–4 hours with at least a 1-hour period of rest on assist/control ventilation in between trials.

     c) Once the patient can breathe spontaneously for approximately 2 hours, extubation is usually considered.

  b. Synchronized intermittent mandatory ventilation

     i. The patient is switched to SIMV mode.

     ii. The RR is reduced to 50%–80% of the baseline rate.

     iii. A CPAP level of up to 5 cm H_2O is preferred by some clinicians.

     iv. The VT and inspiratory flow rate are kept unchanged.

     v. The SIMV rate is decreased by 2–4 breaths/min usually twice per day or more often, depending on the patient's clinical condition.

     vi. If the clinical condition deteriorates, the patient is switched to the assist/control mode of ventilation or, preferably, the preceding rate of SIMV at which the clinical status remained stable.

     vii. Some clinicians prefer to obtain an ABG ½ hour after each ventilator change.

     viii. Once the patient is able to tolerate a ventilator rate of approximately 4 breaths/min for 2 hours without developing respiratory distress, extubation can be considered. Most clinicians will check an ABG before extubation.

     ix. Sometimes in a patient who is able to be weaned, the demand valve on the ventilator may be insensitive, the continuous gas flow may be inadequate for the patient's needs, or delivery of VT may be delayed. The net result may be excessive work of breathing by the patient, even with high ventilator delivery rates. This may result in failure to wean off the SIMV mode.

  c. Pressure support ventilation (PSV)

     i. The initial level of pressure support is generally adjusted to achieve a spontaneous respiratory rate of ≥25 breaths/min. (Usual pressure support level is 10–20 cm H_2O).

     ii. The level of PSV is gradually reduced by 2–4 cm H_2O, usually two to three times per day or more frequently, depending on the patient's clinical condition.

     iii. The RR and clinical condition are closely monitored.

     iv. If the RR increases rapidly or the clinical condition deteriorates when the level of PSV is reduced, the preceding level of pressure support at which the patient's condition was stable should be reverted to.

     v. Patients who are able to tolerate pressure support of approximately 5 cm H_2O for 2 hours without clinical deterioration are extubated, usually after an ABG is checked.

     vi. PSV allows the patient greater autonomy and may theoretically be better tolerated. It may also be used to overcome the imposed airways resistance (e.g., from ET tube, ventilator tubing). (See requisite level of PSV in "Modes of Ventilation" on p 23.)

  d. Combined approaches

     i. PSV may occasionally be combined with SIMV.

     ii. Both may be gradually decreased at the same time, or they may be decreased one at a time (with SIMV usually decreased first).

     iii. There is no specific advantage with this technique in general. It may be part of an ICU protocol designed to overcome a specific problem during weaning.

  e. Role of noninvasive positive pressure ventilation (NIPPV) in weaning

     i. In patients with borderline weaning criteria, a trial of weaning may be undertaken.

     ii. Upon extubation, such patients may be placed on NIPPV, usually for the first 24–48 hours.

     iii. In such instances, an ICU ventilator with a full face mask may be preferable over BiPAP and nasal mask (see section on NIPPV on pp 37–40).

     iv. Using NIPPV as an extension of the weaning process may prevent reintubation in some borderline cases.

  f. Protocol-based weaning

     i. As many as one third of patients who self-extubate do not need to be reintubated. This suggests that weaning may not be done quickly enough in a significant number of mechanically ventilated patients.

     ii. Because weaning is labor intensive in many cases, physicians may not initiate or may abort the process of weaning if they cannot be present to monitor their patients.

   iii. On the other hand, nurses and respiratory therapists may be able to closely monitor the patients during weaning. They could be in-serviced to follow predetermined weaning protocols.

   iv. In a study by Kollef et al (1997), protocol-driven weaning performed by nurses and respiratory therapists was compared with physician-directed weaning. The results are summarized:

	Physician-Directed	Protocol-Driven
• Duration of mechanical ventilation (hours)	102	69*
• Rate of reintubation (%)	10	13
• Cost analysis ($)	27,680	27,439

*P = .029

   v. Thus, predetermined weaning protocols, carried out by appropriately in-serviced nursing and respiratory personnel, may shorten the duration of mechanical ventilation and facilitate weaning.

g. Automatic Weaning Methods

   i. New weaning methods are undergoing trials in which a computer analyzes the patient's lung function and integrates the information with the physician's input (e.g., desired gross V_A) to wean the patient.

   ii. This concept of adaptive lung ventilation is patient centered and takes into consideration several patient breathing-related variables while maintaining a predetermined V_A.

   iii. With such techniques, it is possible for the patient to wean without intervention by a clinician.

   iv. In a recent study, using adaptive lung ventilation controller, 22 out of 27 patients were brought down to an IMV rate of 4 breaths/min and a PSV of 5 cm H_2O within 30 minutes of initiation of the weaning trial. All but one patient was extubated within 24 hours of initiation of trial.

   v. Although it is too early to comment on the usefulness of these techniques, and more information regarding target gross V_A needs to be collected, they may prove to be a safe, rapid, and more physiologic mode of weaning.

h. Other modes of ventilation

   i. Other modes of ventilation that have been tried for weaning include:

     a) Mandatory $\dot{V}_E$

     b) Proportional assist ventilation

F. Comparison of methods of weaning

Different studies have compared different methods of weaning: SIMV, PSV, and spontaneous breathing trials. These studies have reached different conclusions:

1. A prospective trial considered 165 patients randomly assigned to either IMV or T-tube weaning. The duration of time from meeting objective weaning criteria to extubation was 5.3 hours for the IMV group and 5.9 hours for the T-tube group (Tomlinson et al 1989).

2. The mean (±SD) duration of weaning with PSV was 5.7 ± 3.7 days compared with IMV (9.9 ± 8.2 days) and with trials of spontaneous breathing (8.5 ± 8.3 days) (Brochard et al 1994).

3. The once-daily trial of spontaneous breathing led to extubation approximately three times more quickly than SIMV and twice as quickly as PSV (Esteban et al 1995). However, the weaning protocol was more aggressive with a higher rate of reintubation than in Brochard's study (discussed below, in entry 3).

4. A spontaneous breathing trial (on T-tube) was compared with a PSV (7 cm H_2O) trial, each given for 2 hours. Effectiveness of each of the two techniques to predict weaning success was measured at 24 hours after extubation. The success rate was 63% for T-tube and 70% for PSV. Thus, both T-tube and PSV have similar predicted values for weaning success (Esteban et al 1997).

G. Guidelines for weaning (the Medical Intensive Care Unit at Nassau County Medical Center)

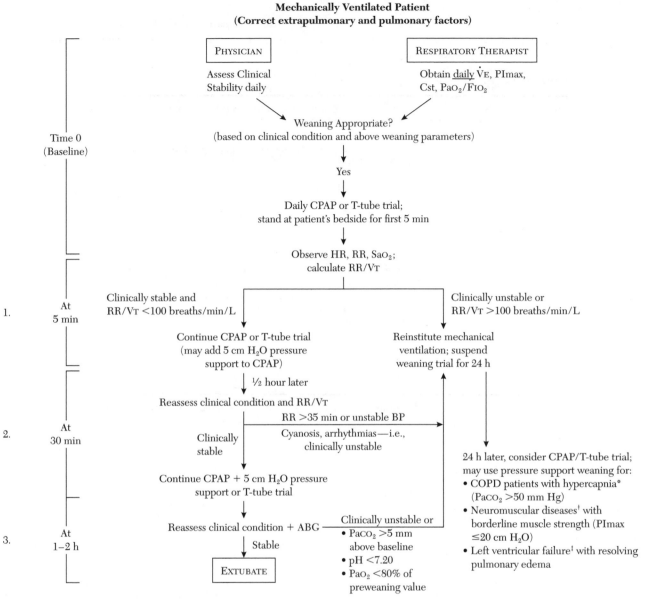

Mechanically Ventilated Patient
(Correct extrapulmonary and pulmonary factors)

PHYSICIAN

Assess Clinical Stability daily

RESPIRATORY THERAPIST

Obtain daily $\dot{V}E$, PImax, Cst, PaO_2/FIO_2

Weaning Appropriate?
(based on clinical condition and above weaning parameters)

Yes

Daily CPAP or T-tube trial; stand at patient's bedside for first 5 min

Observe HR, RR, SaO_2; calculate RR/VT

Time 0 (Baseline)

1. At 5 min

Clinically stable and RR/VT <100 breaths/min/L

Clinically unstable or RR/VT >100 breaths/min/L

Continue CPAP or T-tube trial (may add 5 cm H_2O pressure support to CPAP)

Reinstitute mechanical ventilation; suspend weaning trial for 24 h

½ hour later

Reassess clinical condition and RR/VT

2. At 30 min

RR >35 min or unstable BP
Cyanosis, arrhythmias—i.e., clinically unstable

Clinically stable

24 h later, consider CPAP/T-tube trial; may use pressure support weaning for:
• COPD patients with hypercapnia° ($PaCO_2$ >50 mm Hg)
• Neuromuscular diseases[†] with borderline muscle strength (PImax ≤20 cm H_2O)
• Left ventricular failure[‡] with resolving pulmonary edema

Continue CPAP + 5 cm H_2O pressure support or T-tube trial

3. At 1–2 h

Reassess clinical condition + ABG

Clinically unstable or
• $PaCO_2$ >5 mm above baseline
• pH <7.20
• PaO_2 <80% of preweaning value

Stable

EXTUBATE

° Allow CO_2 to build up slowly to baseline values and for renal compensation to set in.
[†] Slowly build up muscle strength without leading to muscle fatigue.
[‡] Allow diuretics to work and use reduction in venous return by the ventilator in the interim.

H. Extubation protocol guidelines
1. Fulfill predetermined objective criteria for initiating weaning.
2. Choose appropriate time (early in the day).
3. Minimize the use of respiratory depressants. Rarely, in an agitated or apprehensive patient, small doses of anxiolytic agents (e.g., benzodiazepines) may be used.
4. Explain the procedure to the patient.
5. Suction airways as needed.
6. Place the patient in a head-elevated or semi-upright position.
7. Ask the patient to take in a deep breath and to hold it.

8. Deflate tracheal cuff with a syringe and withdraw ET-tube rapidly and smoothly. Ask the patient to exhale.
9. Encourage the patient to cough.
10. Give supplemental oxygen with humidity—for example, with face tent. (F_{IO_2} usually 10% higher than on ventilator.)
11. If clinical condition remains stable, consider getting the patient out of bed to a chair.
12. Incentive spirometry may be useful in some patients who develop atelectasis, have neuromuscular weakness, or are taking rapid, shallow breaths.

I. Parameters to be monitored after extubation

Type of Monitoring	Consider Reconnecting to Ventilator
a. Clinical examination	Diaphoresis
	Increased RR (usually >35 breaths/min), decreased RR (≤ breaths/min), dyspnea
	Paradoxic breathing
	Stridor
	Cyanosis
	Decreased mental status
	Anginal pain
b. Physiologic parameters/ investigations	
ECG	New arrhythmias, ischemia
HR	Tachycardia (HR >100 beats/min), bradycardia (HR <60 beats/min)
BP	Hypertension/hypotension
	Hypotension (mean BP <60 mm Hg or systolic blood pressure <90 mm Hg) or hypertension >170 mm Hg or an increase above baseline >20 mm Hg
RR	Usually >35 breaths/min or ≤6 breaths/min
$\dot{V}_E$	Usually >10 L/min
Pa_{O_2}	<80% preweaning value
Pa_{CO_2}*	>5 mm above baseline
pH*	<7.20

*COPD patients with baseline hypercapnia who develop acute on chronic respiratory acidosis may need to be given noninvasive positive-pressure ventilation or reintubated and mechanically ventilated.

J. Reasons for unsuccessful weaning—an algorithmic approach

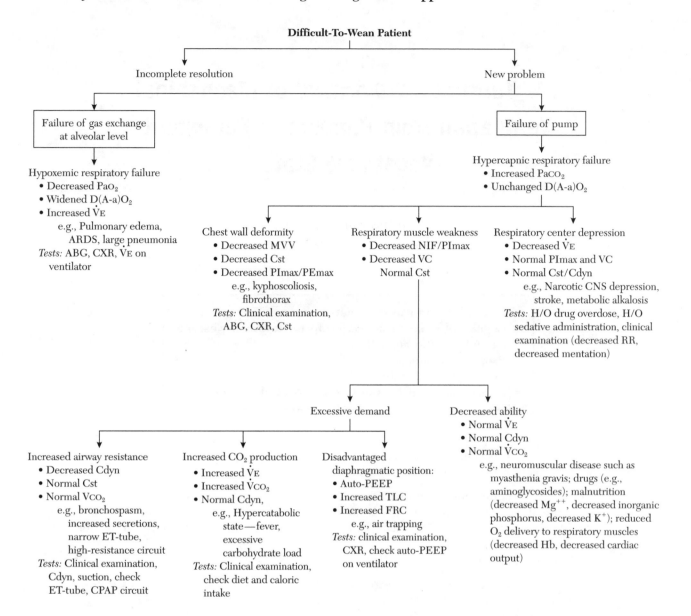

Difficult-To-Wean Patient

Incomplete resolution

New problem

Failure of gas exchange at alveolar level

Failure of pump

Hypoxemic respiratory failure
• Decreased PaO_2
• Widened $D(A-a)O_2$
• Increased $\dot{V}_E$
   e.g., Pulmonary edema, ARDS, large pneumonia
Tests: ABG, CXR, $\dot{V}_E$ on ventilator

Hypercapnic respiratory failure
• Increased $PaCO_2$
• Unchanged $D(A-a)O_2$

Chest wall deformity
• Decreased MVV
• Decreased Cst
• Decreased PImax/PEmax
   e.g., kyphoscoliosis, fibrothorax
Tests: Clinical examination, ABG, CXR, Cst

Respiratory muscle weakness
• Decreased NIF/PImax
• Decreased VC
   Normal Cst

Respiratory center depression
• Decreased $\dot{V}_E$
• Normal PImax and VC
• Normal Cst/Cdyn
   e.g., Narcotic CNS depression, stroke, metabolic alkalosis
Tests: H/O drug overdose, H/O sedative administration, clinical examination (decreased RR, decreased mentation)

Excessive demand

Decreased ability
• Normal $\dot{V}_E$
• Normal Cdyn
• Normal $\dot{V}_{CO_2}$
   e.g., neuromuscular disease such as myasthenia gravis; drugs (e.g., aminoglycosides); malnutrition (decreased Mg^{++}, decreased inorganic phosphorus, decreased K^+); reduced O_2 delivery to respiratory muscles (decreased Hb, decreased cardiac output)

Increased airway resistance
• Decreased Cdyn
• Normal Cst
• Normal $\dot{V}_{CO_2}$
   e.g., bronchospasm, increased secretions, narrow ET-tube, high-resistance circuit
Tests: Clinical examination, Cdyn, suction, check ET-tube, CPAP circuit

Increased CO_2 production
• Increased $\dot{V}_E$
• Increased $\dot{V}_{CO_2}$
• Normal Cdyn,
   e.g., Hypercatabolic state—fever, excessive carbohydrate load
Tests: Clinical examination, check diet and caloric intake

Disadvantaged diaphragmatic position:
• Auto-PEEP
• Increased TLC
• Increased FRC
   e.g., air trapping
Tests: clinical examination, CXR, check auto-PEEP on ventilator

14. Terminal Withdrawal of Mechanical Ventilation from Patients in Persistent Vegetative State

Ashok Karnik, MD

> • Definition and causes of persistent vegetative state
> • Legal and ethical considerations for terminal weaning
> • Guidelines and algorithm
> • Proposed protocol
> • Aftermath of withdrawal
> • Clinical study at Nassau County Medical Center

A. **Introduction**

In the persistent vegetative states, mechanical ventilation may merely prolong existence. Terminal weaning may be considered in such patients.

B. **Definition of persistent vegetative states**
  1. State of chronic wakefulness without awareness
  2. May be accompanied by spontaneous eye opening, brief smiling, instinctive grunts, or screams
  3. Absence of comprehension or coherent speech

C. **Conditions leading to persistent vegetative states at Nassau County Medical Center**
  1. Cerebrovascular accident: 36%
  2. Cardiopulmonary arrest: 23%
  3. Trauma: 18%
  4. Pneumonia: 23%

D. **Legal and ethical considerations in withdrawing ventilatory support**
  1. Authority to consent for withdrawal of mechanical ventilation should be based on clear and convincing evidence that it was the patient's wish not to remain on a ventilator in such a vegetative state. *Clear and convincing evidence would consist of:*
     a. An Advance Directive by the patient.
     b. Decision by a health care proxy who is designated to act on behalf of the patient.
  2. Ethical principles of autonomy, beneficence, and nonmaleficence should be followed.
     a. Autonomy of the patient (i.e., right to refuse treatment) should be respected.
     b. Beneficence and nonmaleficence → life support system should be used only to restore and maintain patient's well-being and not merely to prolong the process of dying.

E. **Guidelines for the withdrawal of life support system**
  1. Follow the general ethical principles of autonomy, beneficence, and nonmaleficence.
  2. Establish the source of authority → patients alone or their legal surrogates have the right to control what happens to them.

3. Clarify prognosis and exercise reasonable clinical judgment regarding the effects of further treatment.
4. Assess the patient's ability/inability to make decisions.
5. Identify any coercive influences, either personal or financial.
6. Keep the discussion of prognosis simple and honest.
7. Explore concurrence of all family members.
8. Allow the family adequate time for decisions.
9. Discuss withdrawal of ventilatory support with the legal department to ensure that a proper and adequate consent is on record.
10. Ensure that there are no disagreements between various health care team members.
11. Withdraw support gradually.
12. Document every assessment, opinion, discussion, and step that leads to actual withdrawal, the detailed observations during the process, and the aftermath.

F. Proposed algorithm for withdrawal of ventilatory support—medical legal aspects.

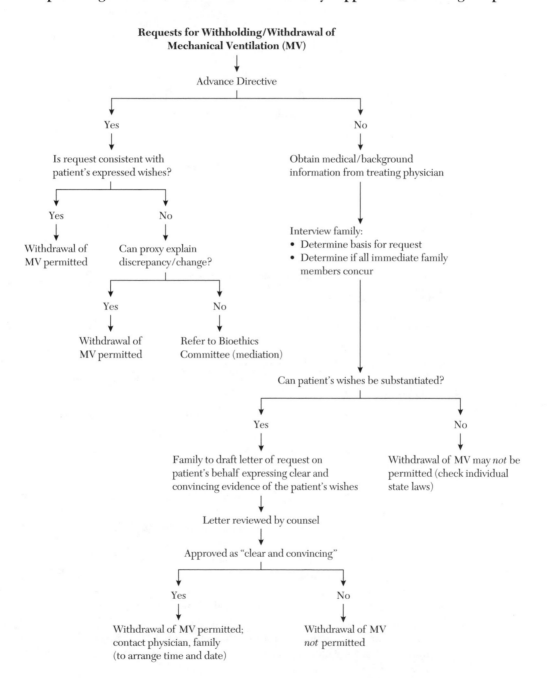

G. Protocol for terminal weaning followed at Nassau County Medical Center

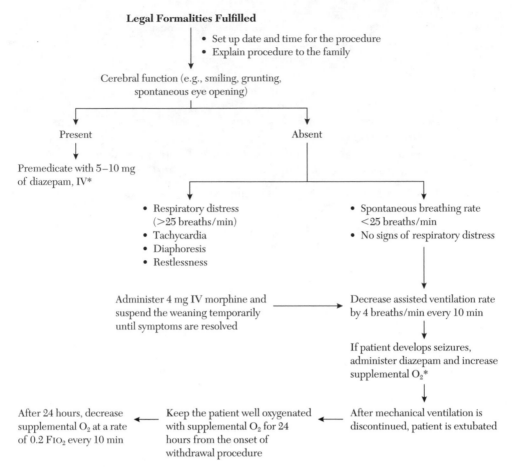

Legal Formalities Fulfilled
- Set up date and time for the procedure
- Explain procedure to the family

Cerebral function (e.g., smiling, grunting, spontaneous eye opening)

Present → Premedicate with 5–10 mg of diazepam, IV*

Absent

- Respiratory distress (>25 breaths/min)
- Tachycardia
- Diaphoresis
- Restlessness

- Spontaneous breathing rate <25 breaths/min
- No signs of respiratory distress

Administer 4 mg IV morphine and suspend the weaning temporarily until symptoms are resolved → Decrease assisted ventilation rate by 4 breaths/min every 10 min

If patient develops seizures, administer diazepam and increase supplemental O_2*

After 24 hours, decrease supplemental O_2 at a rate of 0.2 FIO_2 every 10 min ← Keep the patient well oxygenated with supplemental O_2 for 24 hours from the onset of withdrawal procedure ← After mechanical ventilation is discontinued, patient is extubated

* Morphine or diazepam should be used as needed for patient's comfort and sedation.

H. Aftermath of the withdrawal
1. Death may not occur immediately after withdrawal and a few patients may continue to live for a variable period.
2. It is essential to explain to the family that death is very likely after withdrawal but that the patient may survive for a variable period of time.
3. Prior counseling of the family members helps prevent later expressions of hostility, anger, and complaints against doctors or lawsuits against the hospital.

I. Experience at Nassau County Medical Center on withdrawing ventilatory support in 22 patients in PVS
1. Period of study: July 1991 to December 1994
2. Patient data (n = 22)
   a. Men (n = 10); women (n = 12)
   b. Except for 3 men and 1 woman, all patients were >71 years old at the time of the study
3. Main underlying diagnoses
   a. CVA (n = 8), cardiopulmonary arrest (n = 5), pneumonia (n = 5), trauma (n = 4)
4. Observations
   a. Duration of ventilator therapy: 4–253 days (range).
   b. Institution of mechanical ventilation to the first suggestion regarding withdrawal of ventilatory support (average, 44.4 days).
   c. An average of 16.5 days was required for legal clearance. At present, the period of clearance is significantly shorter.
   d. Most patients had no distressing symptoms during or soon after the withdrawal.
   e. Two "terminally weaned" patients survived and were transferred to a nursing home. They remained in a vegetative state.

III. Problems During Mechanical Ventilation

15. Complications of Mechanical Ventilation

Suhail Allaqaband, MD

> - **Limitations of conventional ventilatory techniques**
> - **Ventilator malfunction**
> - **Adverse effects of excessive pressure and flow rates**
> - **Nosocomial pneumonia**
> - **Hemodynamic effects**
> - **Oxygen toxicity**
> - **Complications of tracheal intubation**
> - **Gastrointestinal complications**
> - **Renal complications**
> - **Nutritional problems**
> - **Psychological trauma**
> - **Side effects of adjuvant drugs**

A. Limitations of conventional ventilation

1. High distending pressures and barotrauma
2. Rapid changes in lung volume → shearing stress on alveoli
3. Hemodynamic compromise
4. Need for intubation (except in noninvasive ventilation)
5. Special problems of oxygenation in severe ARDS and of ventilation in acute, severe asthma and in bronchopleural fistula

B. Ventilator malfunction

1. Machine failure (1.7%)
   a. Causes
      i. Failure to cycle or deliver the set V_T
      ii. Electrical failure or pneumatic failure caused by malfunctioning valves
   b. May lead to hypoxia, hypoventilation, respiratory failure, and death
2. Alarm failure (3.7%)
   a. Caused by inappropriate alarm settings, electrical failure, weak batteries, or being turned off inadvertently
   b. May lead to serious consequences if not noticed in time
3. Inadequate nebulization or humidification (12.7%)
   a. Caused by leaking nebulizer or humidifier, improper placement of nebulizer, no connection with the oxygen source, electrical failure, or improper heat moisturizer exchange (HME)
   b. Inadequate nebulization may result in administration of an improper dosage.
   c. Inadequate humidification may lead to thick secretions and infections (excessive humidification may also contribute to nosocomial infections).

4. Ventilator asynchrony (2%).
    a. Asynchrony between the patient's needs and ventilatory performance is caused by inappropriate ventilator settings (e.g., inappropriate PEEP, flow rate, RR, sensitivity).
    b. Can cause hypoxia, respiratory distress, increased work of breathing.
5. Overheating of inspired air (2%)
    a. Caused by inappropriate ventilator settings, malfunctioning of heater
    b. Can cause thermal injury to the airways
6. Prevention of ventilator malfunction
    a. Proper maintenance of patient ventilator system.
    b. Regular inspection of the equipment.
    c. Patient–ventilator system check should include monitoring patient's response to ventilator.
        i. Checking ventilator alarms, maintaining proper settings.
        ii. Checking ventilator circuit and humidifier (Zwillich et al 1974).
7. Guidelines for ventilator preventive maintenance and remanufacturing followed at Nassau County Medical Center, New York
    a. Puritan Bennett 7200A/AE microprocessor ventilators
        i. Service shall include two scheduled preventive maintenance checks per year.
        ii. Service shall include manufacturer's recommended 2500 hour and 10,000 hour preventive maintenance part kit and procedures for ventilator and internal compressor.
    b. Puritan Bennett MA-1 adult volume ventilator
        i. Service shall include two scheduled preventive maintenance checks per year.
        ii. Per manufacturer's recommendations, MA-1 ventilators will be re-manufactured every 10,000 hours.
    c. Bourns Bear I and II adult volume ventilators
        i. Service shall include three scheduled preventive maintenance checks per year in accordance with the manufacturer's recommendations. Bear I and II ventilators will be re-manufactured every 15,000 hours.
    d. Equipment maintenance
        i. Airdyne air compressors: two preventive maintenance checks per year
        ii. Pediatric aerosol tents: two preventive maintenance checks per year
        iii. Wright or Boehringer Respirometers: two preventive maintenance checks per year
        iv. Bird oxygen blenders: two preventive maintenance checks per year
        v. Oxygen regulators and flow meters: sent out for servicing as needed
    e. Medical gas piping system inspection
        i. Primary medical gas inspection will take place biannually to comply with all JCAHO specifications and guidelines.
        ii. An annual spot inspection shall take place.
    f. Specifications
        i. All equipment shall be completely cleaned and performance tested to ensure that the unit and all subassemblies comply with the manufacturers' specifications.
        ii. Preventive maintenance service will include an electrical safety inspection in accordance with set standards.
        iii. Items attached to the equipment such as heated humidifiers and external flow cables shall be included in the preventive maintenance procedure.
        iv. All equipment shall be recalibrated and recertified. A dated certification sticker shall be attached to each piece of equipment.

C. Adverse effects of excessive pressure and flow rates

Suhail Allaqaband, MD
Suhail Raoof, MD

1. Barotrauma (5%–15%)
   a. Important and potentially lethal complication of mechanical ventilation.
   b. Seen in 4%–15% of patients on mechanical ventilation.
   c. Incidence depends on the underlying lung condition; incidence is highest in ARDS (60%) followed by pneumonia (21%) and COPD (19%).
   d. Mortality is also dependent on underlying pathology: ARDS (60%), non-ARDS (26%).
   e. Barotrauma is most likely to occur if TLC is exceeded. TLC is generally achieved when transalveolar pressures are approximately 30–35 cm H_2O. The closest estimate of transalveolar pressures that can be practically measured is end-inspiratory Pel. This should be kept at <35 cm H_2O.
   f. Barotrauma is more likely to occur with:
   PEEP >15 cm H_2O
   PIP >40–50 cm H_2O (incidence of pneumothorax is 40% if PIP >70 cm H_2O for ≥24 hours). However, these high pressures are generally dissipated in the proximal airways and are usually dampened at the alveolar level.
   V_T >15 mL/kg of body weight
   $\dot{V}_E$ >22 L/min

   g. PIP is a less reliable variable because it may reflect other factors that do not influence alveolar pressure such as flow rate, ET-tube resistance, secretions, and bronchoconstriction. PIP is also affected by increased intra-abdominal pressure (e.g., ascites, ileus, body casts, or tight binder dressings).

High PEEP or
High PIP or ⟶ Forceful leak of gas from the contained airway alveolar complex may cause rupture of alveolar walls adjacent to pulmonary vessels
High tidal volumes

↓

Entry of gas into the perivascular sheath

↓

Proximal dissection into mediastinum

↓

Decompresses through other fascial planes

↓

- Pneumothorax
- Subcutaneous emphysema
- Supleural blebs/cysts
- Pneumopericardium/cardiac tamponade
- Pneumoperitoneum
- Systemic air embolism
- Bronchopleural fistula
- Diffuse lung injury

    h. The possibility of barotrauma can be minimized by:
        i. Keeping transalveolar pressure <30–35 cm H_2O during delivery of each V_T
        ii. Allowing permissive hypercapnia to develop, if needed
        iii. Using pressure control ventilation
        iv. Using $ECCO_2R$ or intracaval gas exchange
        v. High-frequency ventilation
    i. Alveolar overdistension and collapse in ARDS

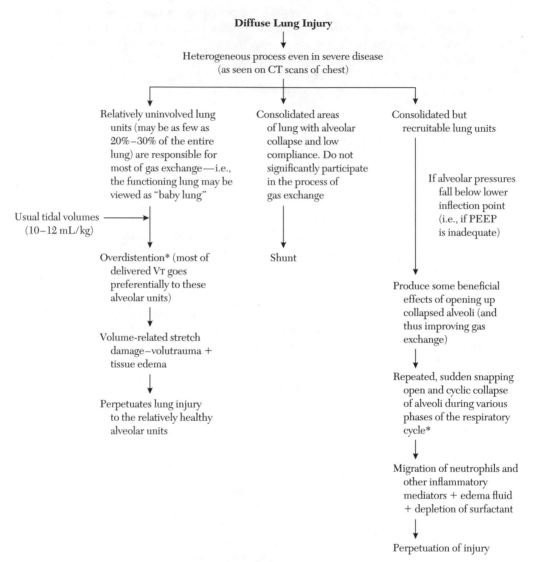

Diffuse Lung Injury

Heterogeneous process even in severe disease
(as seen on CT scans of chest)

Relatively uninvolved lung units (may be as few as 20%–30% of the entire lung) are responsible for most of gas exchange—i.e., the functioning lung may be viewed as "baby lung"

Consolidated areas of lung with alveolar collapse and low compliance. Do not significantly participate in the process of gas exchange

Consolidated but recruitable lung units

Usual tidal volumes (10–12 mL/kg)

If alveolar pressures fall below lower inflection point (i.e., if PEEP is inadequate)

Overdistention* (most of delivered V_T goes preferentially to these alveolar units)

Shunt

Volume-related stretch damage–volutrauma + tissue edema

Produce some beneficial effects of opening up collapsed alveoli (and thus improving gas exchange)

Perpetuates lung injury to the relatively healthy alveolar units

Repeated, sudden snapping open and cyclic collapse of alveoli during various phases of the respiratory cycle*

Migration of neutrophils and other inflammatory mediators + edema fluid + depletion of surfactant

Perpetuation of injury

* These effects may be seen in each of the three populations of alveoli in the ARDS lung.

  2. Volutrauma
    a. Experiments conducted (Dreyfus and colleagues) in ARDS lung model:
        i. Positive-pressure ventilation with large tidal volumes and high inspiratory pressures → acute lung injury
        ii. Negative-pressure ventilation with large tidal volumes and low inspiratory pressures → acute lung injury
        iii. Strap chest wall and ventilate

High pressures   ↓   Low tidal volumes
Minimize lung injury

b. Conclusions
- **OVERDISTENTION, NOT HIGH PRESSURES, LEADS TO LUNG INJURY**
    i. Thus, volume-related alveolar stretch leads to lung injury.
    ii. The more appropriate term is *volutrauma* rather than *barotrauma*.
    iii. In diseases such as ARDS, different populations of alveoli have different levels of static compliance (heterogeneous involvement)

Figure 41

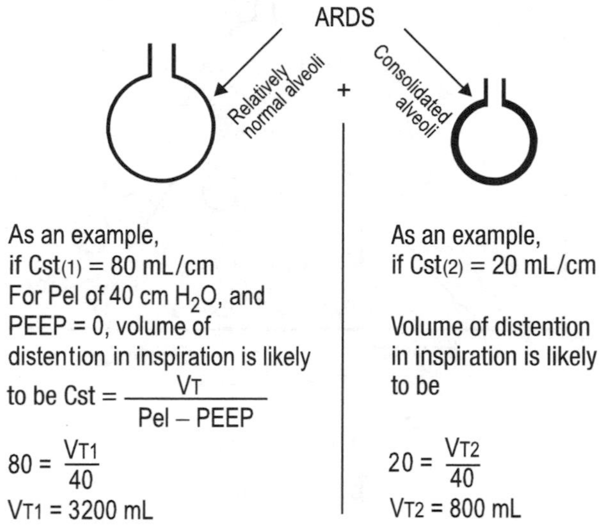

ARDS

Relatively normal alveoli   +   Consolidated alveoli

As an example,
if Cst(1) = 80 mL/cm
For Pel of 40 cm H_2O, and
PEEP = 0, volume of
distention in inspiration is likely

to be Cst = $\dfrac{V_T}{Pel - PEEP}$

$80 = \dfrac{V_{T1}}{40}$

V_{T1} = 3200 mL

As an example,
if Cst(2) = 20 mL/cm

Volume of distention
in inspiration is likely
to be

$20 = \dfrac{V_{T2}}{40}$

V_{T2} = 800 mL

In nonhomogeneous involvement of the lung, the relatively uninvolved populations of alveoli undergo greater distention and are therefore more likely to develop volutrauma.

    iv. Because the volume of the individual alveolus cannot be practically determined, the transalveolar pressure is used as a surrogate. The transalveolar pressure is the difference between the alveolar pressure and the pleural pressure.

Figure 42

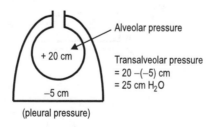

Alveolar pressure

+ 20 cm

Transalveolar pressure
= 20 −(−5) cm
= 25 cm H_2O

−5 cm

(pleural pressure)

    v. Practically, end-inspiratory plateau pressures approximate an average end-inspiratory alveolar pressure.
    vi. A healthy, nonintubated person can develop a transalveolar pressure of only approximately 30 cm H_2O with maximum inspiratory effort.
    vii. A transalveolar pressure of 30 cm H_2O is likely to correspond to an end-inspiratory plateau pressure of 35 cm H_2O.
    viii. Therefore, as a clinical correlate, end-inspiratory plateau pressures of >35 cm H_2O may predict volutrauma.

3. Shear stress: the concept of minimum inflection point
   a. In ARDS, diseased alveoli may collapse during early to mid-exhalation and may open only during mid- to late inspiration.

Figure 43

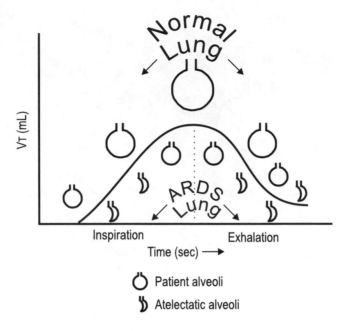

   b. The cyclical opening and closing of alveoli result in a shearing stress that is most profound at the alveolar capillary interface.

Figure 44

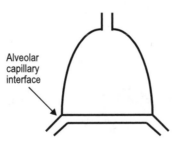

   c. This shearing stress may result in volutrauma.

d. Upper and lower inflection points.

Figure 45

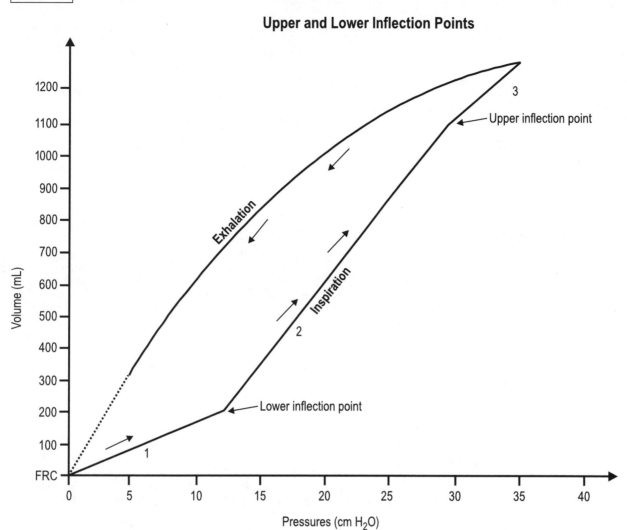

Upper and Lower Inflection Points

Hypothetical depiction of pressure volume curves obtained by passive inflation of lungs using supersyringe technique (see Fig. 18 on p 36)

Phase	Diagram	Description	Implications
I	Volume (mL) 300 / 200 / 100 — Pressure (cm H₂O) 5 10 15 $$Cst(1) = \frac{200}{13} = 15.4 \text{ mL/cm H}_2\text{O}$$	Initial part of pressure-volume curve where many of the alveoli are atelectatic. Hence, static compliance is low—i.e., with a change of 13 cm H_2O of pressure, the change in lung volume is 200 mL.	In this range of operating pressures, a population of alveoli undergoes atelectasis in early to mid-exhalation. Avoid this range of operating pressures to prevent shear stress as alveoli snap open and shut with inspiration and exhalation. Set a level of PEEP that maintains alveolar pressures 1–2 cm H_2O above the lower inflection point—i.e., set PEEP at 14–15 cm H_2O.
II	Volume (mL) 1100 / 200 — Pressure (cm H₂O) 13 30 $$Cst(2) = \frac{\text{change in volume}}{\text{change in pressure}}$$ $$= \frac{1100 - 200}{30 - 13} \text{ mL/cm H}_2\text{O}$$ $$\approx 53 \text{ mL/cm H}_2\text{O}$$	Once the opening pressure or lower inflection point is exceeded, the atelectatic alveoli open. The lung compliance improves—i.e., with a change of pressure of 17 cm H_2O, the change in lung volume is 900 mL.	If the PEEP is set above the opening pressure (lower inflection point), the collapse of alveoli with exhalation is largely prevented. This is likely to reduce large fluctuations in alveolar volume and reduce volutrauma. Oxygenation is likely to improve concomitantly above this point.
III	Volume (mL) 1200 / 1100 — Pressure (cm H₂O) 30 35 $$Cst(3) = \frac{\text{change in volume}}{\text{change in pressure}}$$ $$= \frac{1200 - 1100}{35 - 30} \text{ mL/cm H}_2\text{O}$$ $$= \frac{100}{5} = 20 \text{ mL/cm H}_2\text{O}$$	If the alveoli get overdistended (from either excessive V_T or excessive PEEP), volutrauma, CO_2 retention, and increased pulmonary vascular resistance with extravasation of edema fluid into alveoli are likely to set in. In this phase III, the lung compliance deteriorates—i.e., with a change of 5 cm H_2O of pressure, the change in lung volume is only 100 mL.	The upper inflection point defines the maximal ventilatory pressures recommended. In the example illustrated, the following may be appropriate pressures to set: • PEEP: 14–15 cm H_2O (1–2 cm above lower inflection point) • V_T: up to 900 mL* (below upper inflection point)

* Small V_T so that at the end of the tidal breath, the plateau pressures do not exceed the upper inflection point.

D. Nosocomial pneumonia

Maria Ninivaggi, RN, MSN, CIC
Joanne Selva, RN, BS, CIC

1. Incidence
   a. Seen in 7%–40% patients on mechanical ventilation.
   b. Incidence of pneumonia in intubated, mechanically ventilated patients admitted to the ICU shows a tenfold increase compared with nonventilated patients.
   c. Incidence of nosocomial pneumonia increases with duration of mechanical ventilation.
      i. Five percent in patients on mechanical ventilation for 1 day versus 68.8% in those receiving mechanical ventilation for >30 days
      ii. Mean rate of 1% per day of mechanical ventilation
2. Mortality rate of ventilator-associated pneumonia ranges from 40%–80% in contrast to other patients admitted to the ICU without pneumonia, for whom the mortality rate usually ranges from 2% to 20%.
3. Costs incurred
   a. Nosocomial pneumonia prolongs duration of hospitalization by an average of 9.2 days
4. Causes of nosocomial pneumonias (Data obtained from the Hospital Infectious Program of the CDC: 1986–1994; personal communication)*
   a. *Pseudomonas aeruginosa*   17.9%
   b. *Staphylococcus aureus*   17.4%
   c. *Enterobacter* species   11.5%
   d. *Klebsiella pneumoniae*   6.5%
   e. *Haemophilus influenzae*   5.2%
5. Prevention of nosocomial pneumonia: the basics
   a. Universal precautions and the *consistent* use of personal protective equipment (PPE) are crucial to the prevention of nosocomial infections. Masks and eye covers must be used for procedures likely to generate a spray or splash of body fluids, such as intubation, bronchoscopy, and suctioning. Gloves must be used when procedures are performed such as those listed above, which require direct contact with body fluids. Fluid-impervious gowns are necessary to protect skin/clothing when the above procedures and others that generate spraying or splashing are performed.
   b. Handwashing is the *most critical* factor in the prevention of *all* nosocomial infections among both patients and personnel. Hands must be washed for 10 seconds with an antimicrobial agent before the donning of and upon removal of gloves due to the frequent presence of undetectable holes that permit passage of body fluids and pathogens through the glove barrier. These microscopic holes contribute to contamination of both the patient and the professional.
   c. Aseptic technique (surgical/medical) encompasses the use of thorough hand washing, sterile attire, and maintenance of a sterile field. Preservation of aseptic technique has been shown to be vital in preventing nosocomial infections among critical care patients, who for many reasons have depressed capacity to fight infection.

---

* ICU component of targeted surveillance (85% of patients had ventilator-associated pneumonia)

Specific Prevention of Nosocomial Pneumonia as Related to Risk Factors

Risk Factor	Associated Factors	Prevention Techniques
Nutrition	Enteral tube feeding may increase nasopharyngeal colonization, permit migration of bacteria from the stomach/upper airway, cause reflex/aspiration of gastric contents.	• Discontinue use of enteral feeding tubes as soon as clinically indicated. • When not medically contraindicated, maintain head of bed at 30° to 45° angle to prevent aspiration of stomach contents. • Permit 6- to 8-hour enteral feeding hiatus that facilitates emptying of stomach contents and eliminates neutralizing of gastric secretions. • Periodically monitor placement of the feeding tube. • Assess patient's intestinal motility by auscultating bowel sounds and measuring residual gastric volume or abdominal girth. • Adjust the rate and volume of enteral feedings to avoid regurgitation, in consultation with dietitians. • Fresh enteral feedings should always be provided in clean tubes (tubes must be flushed after feedings). Change tubes according to hospital policy.
Intubation	Ventilator-associated pneumonia (VAP) risk increases 1% per day with intubation due to: • Migration of oropharyngeal organisms via the tube into the trachea • Accumulation of bacteria, over time, on the surface of the tube, forming a biofilm protecting them from antibiotics	• Remove tube when no longer medically indicated. • Technique of insertion should be clean. • Provide gentle suction of secretions using sterile single-use catheter for each series of suctioning or in-line sheath protected suction catheter changed every 24 hours. • Assist secretion drainage by positioning patient with head of bed at 30°–45°. • Drain and discard condensate from inspiratory tubing; do not permit drainage back into patient. • Drain condensate into container appropriate for that use, check hospital policy. • Use of self-contained suctioning devices such as Ballard system decreases risk of infections by avoiding repeated opening of the ventilator tubing during suctioning.
	Pooled subglottic secretions.	• Collection of secretions above the cuff of endotracheal or tracheostomy tube is a major reservoir for infectious agents. Continuous suctioning of this space has been shown to reduce the development of nosocomial pneumonia in chronically ventilated patients. Advantages: • Significant decrease in nosocomial VAP secondary to gram-positive cocci and *Haemophilus influenzae*. • Cost effective and simple. • Reduces therapeutic antibiotic dosing for VAP. Disadvantages: • Does not affect reduction of VAP caused by Enterobacteriaceae or *Pseudomonas aeruginosa*. • Vigilant cuff pressure monitoring by staff is required.
Immobility	Prolonged immobility contributes to stasis of secretions and decreased lung expansion.	• Discontinue mechanical ventilation when medically indicated. • Consider upright sitting in bed or chair as soon as possible. May also consider use of kinetic therapy (specialty beds), if indicated.

Risk Factor	Associated Factors	Prevention Techniques
Impaired consciousness	Combines risks of immobility and depressed or absent gag reflex with the invasive device of intubation.	• If condition is medically induced, cease administration of CNS depressants as soon as medically indicated. • If medically feasible, maintain head of bed at 30°–45° angle to prevent aspiration of stomach contents.
Epidemiologically significant pathogens	Recent antibiotic susceptibility trends have elucidated several virtually untreatable organisms.	• Vancomycin-resistant enterococcus (VRE), unlike other multidrug resistant organisms, is highly associated with the environment for its transmission. Patient and equipment must be isolated; check hospital policy. • Multidrug-resistant tuberculosis (MDR-TB) and tuberculosis should be considered in patients presenting with pulmonary conditions and those with HIV. Early identification and respiratory isolation are indicated. • Methicillin-resistant *Staphylococcus aureus* and resistant *Staphylococcus epidermidis*: use contact isolation and cohorting of patients. • Gram-negative pathogens: give astute priority to technique. Use contact isolation and cohorting of patients.
Gastric colonization	Gastric bacterial burden increases the potential for infection.	• Stress ulcer prophylaxis should be considered only in patients at high risk for GI bleed (prior peptic ulcer disease or UGI bleeding, mechanically ventilated patients, steriod usage and head injury). • Early nutritional enteric support is useful for prevention of stress or gastric ulcers. • CDC guidelines (1994): No recommendation for route acidification of gastric feedings to prevent nosocomial pneumonia.

E. Hemodynamic effects associated with mechanical ventilation
Suhail Allaqaband, MD

1. Hemodynamic effects are mainly caused by changes in *lung volume* and *intrathoracic pressure*.
2. Changes in lung volume lead to vagally mediated reflex arcs, which will cause the heart rate to decrease and result in arterial vasodilatation.
3. Both increased lung volume and increased intrathoracic pressure → increased pulmonary vascular resistance → increased right ventricular end diastolic volume → shift of interventricular septum towards the left ventricle → decreased left ventricular diastolic compliance and decreased contractility.
4. Increased pulmonary venous pressure also leads to increased lung water and increased interstitial–alveolar edema.
5. Increased intrathoracic pressure causes compression of the superior and inferior vena cava, which decreases the venous return and thus the right ventricular filling, leading to decreased cardiac output, decreased arterial blood pressure, and increased systemic venous pressure.
6. Mechanical ventilation increases right ventricular afterload by compressing the pulmonary vessels. The increased right ventricular afterload may cause tricuspid regurgitation.
7. Life-threatening hypotension may occur during the first 2 hours after intubation, particularly if associated with hypovolemia.
8. Effect of mechanical ventilation on cardiac function (especially in hypovolemic states).

Figure 46

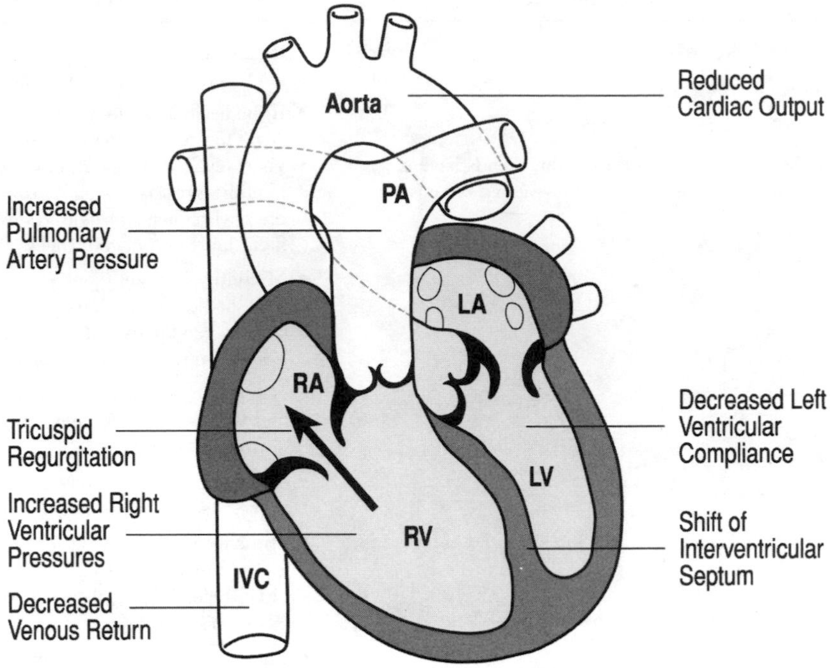

9. Effects of various ventilator modes on cardiovascular system
   a. Spontaneous ventilation
      i. Best in hypovolemic patients because venous return is augmented with each breath.
      ii. Inspiratory negative swings in pleural pressure are increased in conditions like acute asthma, upper airways obstruction, or decreased lung compliance, which leads to decreased cardiac output caused by increased left ventricular afterload.
      iii. Decreased pleural pressure may also decrease pulmonary interstitial pressure, which leads to increased extravascular lung water content.
   b. Assist/control mode ventilation
      i. May be associated with high $\overline{Paw}$ as each spontaneous breath triggers a mechanical one, which may have serious adverse consequences on the cardiovascular system (this is especially true if patient generates rapid RRs).
      ii. Respiratory alkalosis can occur, which can lead to hypokalemia and arrhythmias
   c. Synchronized intermittent mode ventilation
      i. Supplements patient's spontaneous breathing
      ii. Negative intrapleural pressure during spontaneous breathing produces lower $\overline{Paw}$ that is beneficial to the cardiovascular system
   d. Positive end-expiratory pressure/continuous positive airways pressure
      i. Increases airway pressure continuously.
      ii. Increased PEEP leads to decreased cardiac output.
      iii. PEEP beneficial in cardiogenic pulmonary edema as it decreases both preload and afterload improves oxygenation, and decreases work of breathing.
   e. Inverse ratio ventilation
      i. High $\overline{Paw}$ as intrathoracic pressure is increased during most of the respiratory cycle leading to a considerable decrease in cardiac output.

F. Oxygen toxicity (FIO_2 >60% for >4–5 days)

1. Respiratory effects
   a. Depression of respiratory drive
      i. Hypoxic ventilatory drive
      ii. Haldane effect: higher concentration of Hb with oxygen → less CO_2 carried in the blood for the same PCO_2 → increase in tissue PCO_2.

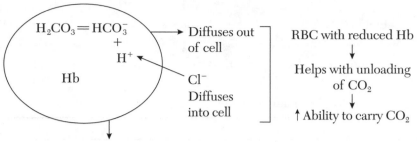

Higher concentration of Hb with oxygen (HbO$_2$)

Oxygenated Hb is more acidic

Helps with unloading of CO$_2$ (less CO$_2$ carried in blood for same PCO$_2$)

Increase in tissue PCO$_2$

      iii. Decreased ventilation/perfusion matching (increased PaO$_2$, loss of hypoxic pulmonary vasoconstriction)
      iv. Reabsorptive atelectasis
  b. Pulmonary vasodilation
  c. Acute tracheobronchitis
  d. Impaired mucociliary clearance
  e. Diffuse alveolar damage (ARDS-like picture)
  f. Bronchopulmonary dysplasia (following therapy for infant respiratory distress syndrome in newborn)
2. Nonrespiratory effects
  a. Hemodynamic changes (decreased HR, decreased cardiac output, decreased $\overline{PAP}$, increased SVR)
  b. Suppressed erythropoiesis
  c. Retrolental fibroplasia of the newborn
3. Mechanism of toxicity

$$O_2 \xrightarrow[2H^+]{e^-} \underset{\text{dismutase}}{O_2 \text{ superoxide}} \xrightarrow[\text{glutathione reductase}]{(-)} H_2O_2 \xrightarrow[\text{catalase}]{e^- + H^+} OH^- + H_2O$$

where
    O$_2$ = superoxide radical   (High reactivity of intermediate free radicals)
    H$_2$O$_2$ = hydrogen peroxide
    OH$^-$ = hydroxyl radical

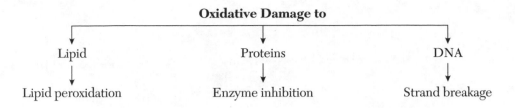

Oxidative Damage to

Lipid	Proteins	DNA
↓	↓	↓
Lipid peroxidation	Enzyme inhibition	Strand breakage

4. Stages of toxicity (0.8–1 atm of oxygen)*

Changes	Time
1. Exudative	Week 1
a. Capillary congestion	3 d
b. Interstitial edema	3 d
c. Hyaline membrane formation	1–7 d
2. Proliferative	After Week 1
a. Alveolar lining cell hyperplasia	1 wk
b. Destruction of type I epithelial cells and proliferation of type II epithelial cells	1 wk
c. Interstitial fibrosis	1–2 wk
d. Pleural effusions	1 wk

* Adapted with permission from Balantine JD. Pathology of Oxygen Toxicity. New York: Academic Press; 1982:116.

5. Safe F_{IO_2} concentration
   a. 50% oxygen: "safe" limit for prolonged exposure
   b. 80% oxygen: relatively "safe" for ≥48 hours
   c. 100% oxygen: relatively "safe" for up to 2 days (some damage within 24 hours)
6. Diagnosis
   a. History of oxygen administration > 0.50–0.60 × 48 hours
   b. Retrosternal pain (acute tracheobronchitis)
   c. Decreasing vital capacity
   d. Radiographically evident diffuse alveolar damage (usually after 60 hours of 1.0 F_{IO_2}) (indistinguishable from ARDS)
7. Management
   a. Lowest F_{IO_2} to obtain an SaO_2 of 90%
   b. PEEP therapy (for diffuse alveolar damage) to lower F_{IO_2}
   c. Minimize excess oxygen demands (e.g., treat fever)
   d. Improve oxygen delivery (increase Hct, increase CO):

$$DO_2 = CO \times CaO_2$$

   where

   DO_2 = oxygen delivery (oxygen transport)
   CO = cardiac output
   CaO_2 = arterial oxygen content

   and

$$CaO_2 = 1.34 \times Hb \times SaO_2 + 0.003 \times PaO_2$$

   where

   Hb = hemoglobin concentration
   SaO_2 = arterial oxygen saturation
   PaO_2 = partial pressure for oxygen in arterial blood

   e. Experimental therapy: e.g., ascorbic acid, β-carotenes, glutathione, surfactant
8. Clinical pearls
   a. The risks of prolonged hypoxia are more serious than the risks of hyperoxia.
   b. Hyperoxic injury can also be produced by the *herbicide* paraquat, *chemotherapeutic agents,* such as bleomycin and mitomycin, and *antimicrobials,* such as nitrofurantoin.

    c. In patients who have received agents such as bleomycin, pulmonary toxicity may be precipitated by an $F_{IO_2} \geq 0.3$. Toxicity may occur within 24–72 hours if bleomycin was administered during the last 6 months.

    d. Lung injury mediated by hyperoxia may be almost completely reversible.

    e. The presence of underlying lung disease or mechanical ventilation may increase the sensitivity of oxygen toxicity.

    f. Pre-exposure to sublethal levels of hyperoxia or endotoxin in some species may induce antioxidant enzyme levels and increase resistance to hyperoxic lung injury. Surfactant may play a protective role.

    g. Nutritional deficiencies (e.g., vitamins E and C and selenium) may decrease antioxidants and potentiate hyperoxic lung injury.

G. Complications of tracheal intubation

1. Local airway damage
   a. Tracheal, nasal, paranasal, and laryngeal inflammation
   b. Vocal cord paralysis
   c. Tracheal stenosis
   d. Granuloma
   e. Tracheomalacia
2. Airway colonization → nosocomial pneumonia

H. Gastrointestinal complications

1. Gastrointestinal bleed
   a. Incidence >40% in patients who are on mechanical ventilation for >3 days
   b. ↑ Intrathoracic pressure → decreased cardiac output and increased venous pressure → ischemia of gastrointestinal mucosa → ulceration → bleeding
   c. May be prevented in some cases by using sucralfate or H_2 blockers prophylactically
2. Meteorism
   a. Massive gastric distention caused by inspiratory gas leaking around the endotracheal tube cuff
   b. Can lead to gastric rupture
   c. Prevented or alleviated by the passage of a small-bore nasogastric tube
3. Gastroduodenal dysfunction
4. Gastrointestinal colonization by gram-negative bacilli

I. Renal complications

↑ intrathoracic pressure → decreased right ventricular filling → decreased cardiac output → decreased arterial pressure → decreased renal blood flow → increased renin-angiotensin-aldosterone, increased antidiuretic hormone, decreased atrial natriuretic factor → decreased urine volume

J. Nutritional problems

1. Increased caloric requirements due to the hypercatabolic state
2. Increased $PaCO_2$ due to increased carbohydrate load

K. Psychological trauma

1. Some patients perceive mechanical ventilation as "resuscitation with every breath."
2. Some develop feelings of insecurity, fear, and anxiety.
3. Some fear never being able to get off the ventilator; others fear getting off the ventilator and not being able to breathe spontaneously.

L. Side effects of adjuvant drugs

1. Drugs such as morphine, benzodiazepines, and some neuromuscular blockers may be used in patients on mechanical ventilation.
2. These drugs can lead to cardiovascular and CNS depression.
3. Cardiovascular depression may lead to decreased BP, decreased cardiac output, and decreased left ventricular stroke volume.

16. Special Problems with Mechanical Ventilation in Different Clinical Settings

Suhail Raoof, MD

> - **Acute asthma**
> - **Chronic obstructive pulmonary disease**
> - **Adult respiratory distress syndrome**
> - **Cerebrovascular accidents**

A. Acute asthma

Problem	Physiologic Basis	Detection	Solution
1. Hypotension	a. Auto-PEEP Bronchospasm ↓ Air trapping ↓ Decreased venous return ↓ Decreased cardiac output	Monitor airway pressures at end exhalation after closing the exhalation port.	1. Small V_T (10 mL/kg) and low $\dot{V}_E$. 2. Highest peak inspiratory flows (approximately 80 L/min)* that will not cause PIPs to exceed 35–40 cm H_2O. 3. Bronchodilators. 4. Sedate or paralyze, if necessary. 5. PEEP therapy (a few centimeters less than auto-PEEP). 6. Orotracheal intubation (not nasotracheal) with ET-tube size >8. 7. Remove resistance from ventilator circuit (Edith valve, secretions). Use low compressible volume circuit. 8. Fluid resuscitation. 9. Right-heart catheter with administration of pressors, if neccessary.
	b. Pneumothorax High peak pressures	Chest radiograph Increased peak inspiratory and plateau pressures	1. Chest tube insertion. 2. Lowered $\dot{V}_E$. 3. Sedation. 4. Bronchodilators.
	c. Right main stem branches intubation Increased PIPs ↓ Decreased venous return ↓ Decreased cardiac output	Auscultation Chest radiograph	1. Pull back tube. 2. Secure ET-tube. 3. Sedation, if needed.
	d. Dehydration	Decrease in BP soon after intubation	1. Empiric fluid challenge. 2. Right-heart catheter, if necessary.

* Before sedating, ensure that there is no pathologic reason for the restlessness (e.g., hypoxemia, low peak inspiratory flows).

(continues)

A. Acute asthma—cont'd

Problem	Physiologic Basis	Detection	Solution
	e. Sedatives or narcotics (benzodiazepines or morphine)	Decrease in BP soon after administration of medication	1. Naloxone (if morphine was used). Usual dose: 0.4–2 mg IV, repeat every 2 min until a maximum of 10 mg is given. To start a drip, add 2 mg naloxone in 500 mL of D_5W or NS and titrate to patient response. 2. Flumazenil (if benzodiazepine was used. Flumazenil generally does not reverse hypotension but antagonizes excessive sedation and impaired psychomotor recall). 3. Fluid resuscitation.
2. High peak inspiratory pressures	a. Bronchospasm	1. High PIP, normal Pel 2. Check airway resistance: $$\frac{PIP - Pel}{Peak\ insp\ flow} > 10\ cm\ H_2O/L/sec$$	1. Decrease $\dot{V}_E$. 2. Decrease peak inspiratory flows. 3. Sedate ± paralyze.
	b. Auto-PEEP	As above—1(a)	As above—1(a)
	c. Pneumothorax	1. Increased PIP 2. Increased Pel 3. Absent breath sounds 4. CXR	As above—1(b).
	d. Right main stem intubation	1. Increased PIP 2. Increased Pel 3. Decreased breath sounds 4. CXR 5. ET-tube marking shows tube too far in	As above—1(c).
	e. Secretions ± atelectasis	Increased PIP (Pel normal, unless lobar atelectasis)	1. Percussion therapy. 2. Directional suctioning. 3. Bronchodilators (β_2 agonists, ± low-dose theophylline) 4. ± Bronchoscopy.
	f. Patient–ventilator dysynchrony	1. Observe patient: Under ventilated or no sighs	1. Administer manually triggered tidal volumes at rate faster than patient's spontaneous rate, until patient stops making respiratory efforts. 2. Monitor airway pressures and BP. 3. Then titrate $\dot{V}_E$ to lower levels (once work of breathing, oxygen, and $\dot{V}_{O_2}$ are reduced, it is typical to establish a lower $\dot{V}_E$ different from original ventilator settings).

(*continues*)

A. Acute asthma—cont'd

Problem	Physiologic Basis	Detection	Solution
High peak inspiratory fighting pressures—cont'd		2. Pain 3. ET-tube irritating airways 4. Anxiety	• Analgesics. • Topical lidocaine spray. • Sedatives.*
3. Increasing hypercapnia	a. Bronchospasm (inability to ventilate)	1. Auscultation (rhonchi, air entry decreased, i.e., silent chest) 2. Increased PIP and normal Pel	1. Bronchodilators. 2. Sedate ± paralyze. 3. Permissive hypercapnia. 4. Heliox mixture (specific ventilators only)
	b. Hypotension Decreased BP ↓ Decreased cardiac output ↓ Decreased pulmonary blood flow ↓ Increased dead space ↓ Ineffective CO_2 removal	Low BP	1. Fluids. 2. ± Pressors.
	c. Patient–ventilator dysynchrony Decreased effective $\dot{V}_E$	As above—2(f)	As above—2(f).
	d. Permissive hypercapnia	Low $\dot{V}_E$	Acceptable management strategy (see pp 41–43).
	e. Large pulmonary embolism ↓ Dead space ventilation ↓ Sedated patient may not be able to increase $\dot{V}_E$	$\dot{V}/\dot{Q}$ scan Normal PIP and normal Pel	Anticoagulation.
4. Severe hypoxemia (See p 110 for further discussion)	a. Pneumothorax	As above—1(b)	As above—1(b).
	b. (R) Main stem intubation	As above—1(c)	As above—1(c).
	c. Atelectasis	As above—2(e)	As above—2(e).
	d. Severe $\dot{V}/\dot{Q}$ mismatch	1. Wheezing 2. Increased PIP; normal Pel	As above—2(a).
	e. Pneumonia	Chest radiograph	Antibiotics.
	f. Frequent suctioning	Increased secretions; history of frequent suctioning	Limit suctioning. Indwelling suction catheter.
	g. Aspiration	Chest radiograph	Antibiotics, NGT, suction.
	h. Pulmonary embolism	PIP and normal Pel; $\dot{V}/\dot{Q}$ scan abnormal	Anticoagulation.

* Before sedating, ensure that there is no pathologic reason for the restlessness (e.g., hypoxemia, low peak inspiratory flows).

B. Chronic obstructive pulmonary disease (all problems as seen in acute asthmatics)

Problem	Physiologic Basis	Detection	Solution
1. Posthyper-capnic metabolic alkalosis (may result in tetany and seizures)	a. Normalizing arterial $PaCO_2$ (in patients with chronic CO_2 retention)	pH (>7.50) Usually $PaCO_2$ is below patient's baseline value	1. Lower $\dot{V}E$ to normalize pH. 2. Replenish chloride ions (via normal saline infusion) to allow HCO_3 excretion; preferable to administer KCl if patient is hypokalemic. 3. Acetazolamide (specific situations).
	b. Hyperventilation (pain, anxiety)	As above—1(a)	1. Pain relief, sedation. 2. Consider switching to IMV mode with adequate $\dot{V}E$.

C. Adult respiratory distress syndrome

Problem	Physiologic Basis	Detection	Solution
1. Refractory hypoxemia	a. Severe $\dot{V}/\dot{Q}$ mismatch, (shunt) b. Oxygen toxicity c. Rule out barotrauma or volutrauma d. Rule out volume overload	Decreased PaO_2 on ABG	1. Increase FIO_2 if $SaO_2 < 85\%$–87%. 2. Optimize PEEP therapy. (Determine lower inflection point, if possible.) 3. Optimize PAOP. 4. Sedate $\pm$ paralyze. 5. Prolong inspiratory time ($\pm$ pressure control) 6. Prone position ventilation. 7. Nitric oxide. 8. High-frequency ventilation. 9. Experimental therapy: ECMO, oxygen insufflation directly into blood (IVOX), surfactant therapy.
2. High PIP and Pel	Stiff lungs $\rightarrow$ increased pressures	1. Increased PIP Increased Pel 2. Bilateral diffuse alveolar process on chest radiograph	1. Decreased VT, decreased $\dot{V}E$ (permissive hypercapnia). 2. Lower peak inspiratory flows (monitor patient's intrinsic inspiratory flows, SaO_2). 3. Sedate, $\pm$ paralyze. 4. Pressure control ventilation. 5. High-frequency ventilation.
3. Hypotension	Auto-PEEP $\dot{V}E$ (>15 L) $\downarrow$ Air trapping • Pneumothorax • (R) Main stem intubation • Dehydration • Sedatives	$\dot{V}E$ requirements high ($+$) pressures at end expiration As with asthma 1(b) (p 104) As with asthma 1(c) (p 104) As with asthma 1(d) (p 104) As with asthma 1(e) (p 105)	As with asthma 1(a) (p 104) As with asthma 1(b) (p 104) As with asthma 1(c) (p 104) As with asthma 1(d) (p 104) As with asthma 1(e) (p 105)

(continues)

C. Adult respiratory distress syndrome—cont'd

Problem	Physiologic Basis	Detection	Solution
4. Cuff leaks	a. Cuff rupture	• Low exhaled V_T and low-pressure alarms sounding	• Change ET-tube
	b. Malposition of ET-tube	• Check ET-tube position on CXR	• Reposition ET-tube
	c. Leak of pilot balloon	• Check CXR for pilot balloon leak (assess volume of leak: inspired volume − exhaled volume)	• Either reintubate or accept air leak (↑ V_T; monitor $PaCO_2$)
	d. Development of tracheomalacia	• Introduce air, check if cuff leak stops	• Either reintubate or accept air leak (↑ V_T; monitor $PaCO_2$)
5. Tracheomalacia	Cuff overdistended: High airway pressures ↓ Air leak ↓ More air put in cuff ↓ Tracheal mucosal damage	CXR (Cuff:trachea::>1.5:1)	1. Change body position (to minimize leak). 2. Change site of cuff. (Special ET-tubes that are longer may be needed.) 3. Keep cuff pressures <20 mm Hg in most cases. 4. Rarely, pressures between 20 and 25 mm Hg may be needed.
6. Bronchopleural fistula	Persistent leak caused by high pressures: Increased Pel ↓ Alveolar damage ↓ Volutrauma	Persistent air leak detected >3 d after pneumothorax	1. Decreased $\dot{V}_E$. 2. V_T approximately 5–7 mL/kg, if possible. 3. Minimize PEEP. 4. Chest tube PEEP. 5. Minimize inspiratory time (lower I:E ratio). 6. Minimize chest tube suction. 7. Sedate + paralyze. 8. IMV (low rate) + PSV. 9. Independent lung ventilation. 10. High-frequency ventilation.

D. Cerebrovascular accidents (strokes)

Problem	Physiologic Basis	Detection	Solution
1. Severe respiratory alkalosis*	Hyperventilation (unstable respiratory drive)	Decreased $PaCO_2$ Increasing pH Increased RR and $\dot{V}_E$	Sedation (may interfere with clinical evaluation in acute stages) Switch to IMV mode with adequate $\dot{V}_E$*
2. Acute respiratory acidosis*	Hypoventilation acutely (changing respiratory drive)	Increased $PaCO_2$ Decreasing pH Increased RR and $\dot{V}_E$	Back-up rate (A/C or IMV) should be sufficient to ensure adequate ventilation (if spontaneous drive were to cease)

* It may be appropriate to keep patients with CNS disorders who hyperventilate on IMV mode with adequate back-up $\dot{V}_E$.

17. Troubleshooting on Mechanical Ventilation

Faroque A. Khan, MB, and Suhail Raoof, MD

- **Patient-ventilator dysynchrony**
- **Alarms sounding**
- **Hypoxemia**

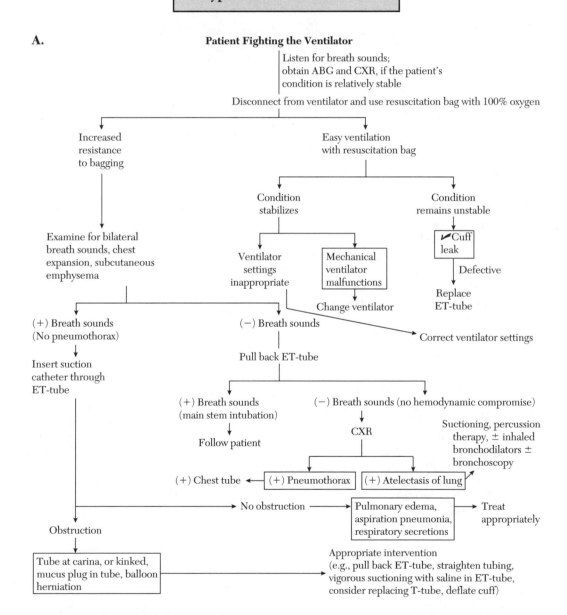

A. **Patient Fighting the Ventilator**

Listen for breath sounds; obtain ABG and CXR, if the patient's condition is relatively stable

Disconnect from ventilator and use resuscitation bag with 100% oxygen

Increased resistance to bagging

Easy ventilation with resuscitation bag

Condition stabilizes

Condition remains unstable

Examine for bilateral breath sounds, chest expansion, subcutaneous emphysema

Ventilator settings inappropriate

Mechanical ventilator malfunctions

✔Cuff leak

Defective

Change ventilator

Replace ET-tube

(+) Breath sounds (No pneumothorax)

(−) Breath sounds

Correct ventilator settings

Insert suction catheter through ET-tube

Pull back ET-tube

(+) Breath sounds (main stem intubation)

(−) Breath sounds (no hemodynamic compromise)

Suctioning, percussion therapy, ± inhaled bronchodilators ± bronchoscopy

Follow patient

CXR

(+) Chest tube ◄— (+) Pneumothorax | (+) Atelectasis of lung

No obstruction

Pulmonary edema, aspiration pneumonia, respiratory secretions

Treat appropriately

Obstruction

Tube at carina, or kinked, mucus plug in tube, balloon herniation

Appropriate intervention (e.g., pull back ET-tube, straighten tubing, vigorous suctioning with saline in ET-tube, consider replacing T-tube, deflate cuff)

B.

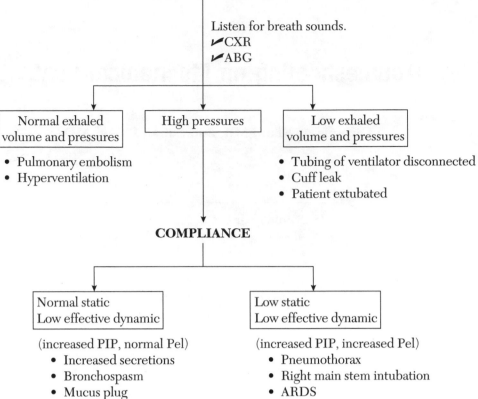

Ventilator Alarms Go Off

Listen for breath sounds.
✔CXR
✔ABG

Normal exhaled volume and pressures	High pressures	Low exhaled volume and pressures
• Pulmonary embolism • Hyperventilation		• Tubing of ventilator disconnected • Cuff leak • Patient extubated

COMPLIANCE

Normal static Low effective dynamic	Low static Low effective dynamic
(increased PIP, normal Pel) • Increased secretions • Bronchospasm • Mucus plug • Tube kinked or occluded	(increased PIP, increased Pel) • Pneumothorax • Right main stem intubation • ARDS • Lobar atelectasis

C. Hypoxemia
(Reprinted with permission from Glauser FL, Polatty RC, Sessler CN. Worsening oxygenation in mechanically ventilated patients. Am Rev Respir Dis. 1988;138:458-65).
1. Ventilator-related problems
   a. ET-tube/tracheostomy malfunction
   b. Improper ventilator settings
   c. Ventilator malfunction
2. Progression of underlying disease process
   a. ARDS
   b. Cardiogenic pulmonary edema
   c. Pneumonia
   d. Airways obstruction (COPD/asthma)
3. New problem
   a. Pneumothorax
   b. Lobar atelectasis
   c. Gastric aspiration
   d. Nosocomial pneumonia
   e. Pulmonary emboli
   f. Fluid overload
   g. Microatelectasis
   h. Bronchospasm
   i. Retained secretions

4. Interventions
   a. ET-tube suctioning
   b. Position changes
   c. Chest percussion therapy
   d. Bronchoscopy
5. Medications
   a. Bronchodilators
   b. Vasodilators
6. Spurious hypoxemia
   a. Hyperthermia
   b. Delay in transport of sample
   c. Leukocyte larceny

18. Nutrition in Mechanically Ventilated Patients

Christos P. Carvounis, MD

> - **Causes of increased nutritional requirements**
> - **Clinical significance of malnutrition**
> - **Role of nutritional repletion in malnourished states**
> - **Disorders of nutrition**
> - **Assessment of nutritional status in mechanically ventilated patients**
> - **Principles of nutritional therapy**
> - **Selection of nutritional prescription**

A. **Nature of the problem**
   1. Oral feeding is difficult.
   2. Starvation has few short-term consequences but worsens outcome and increases mortality in the long run.
   3. Overfeeding, especially with carbohydrates, may result in increased $\dot{V}CO_2$, culminating in greater values of $\dot{V}E$ and failure to wean.

$$V_A = \frac{(K)\dot{V}CO_2}{PaCO_2}$$

   Thus, $\dot{V}A$ is directly proportional to $\dot{V}CO_2$

B. **Causes of increased nutritional requirements in mechanically ventilated patients**
   1. Increased caloric demands
      a. Greater work of breathing
      b. Sepsis
      c. Fever
      d. Wound healing
      e. Hormone release
   2. Decreased caloric intake
   3. Decreased bowel and liver perfusion
   4. Multiple organ failure
   5. Medications
   6. Compromised initial nutritional status

C. **Clinical significance of malnutrition**
   1. Host defenses
      a. Impaired immune response. Mainly T-cell, but also B-cell, dysfunction.
      b. Liver mass decreases. Diminished acute phase reactants and visceral proteins.
   2. Respiratory system
      a. Decreased diaphragmatic muscle mass
      b. Reduction of ventilatory drive
      c. Lung parenchymal changes (loss of elastic fibers, decreased surfactant production)

D. Role of nutritional repletion in malnourished states

1. In patients with acute illness, nutritional repletion probably improves patient outcome (Grote et al 1987; Mullen et al 1980; Wilmore 1983).
2. In unstressed patients, there is no effect on complication rate or survival.

E. Disorders of nutrition (two major syndromes)

1. Marasmus
   a. Produced by long-term decreased caloric intake over weeks to months, such as in starvation malignancy or AIDS.
   b. Dominant characteristics: decreased somatic proteins (muscle) often recognized by temporal wasting; loss of fat (weight loss).
   c. Decreased muscular function including the respiratory muscles is a major problem.
   d. A mechanically ventilated patient may be difficult to wean off a respirator and may require long-term nutritional repletion.
   e. Long-term calorie depletion has produced some significant metabolic disorders (e.g., intracellular phosphorus may be quite low—much lower than indicated by an almost normal blood phosphorus level).
   f. If sugar is given rapidly and to a significant amount, insulin production results that in turn causes glucose to enter the cells. Glucose metabolism (glycolysis) eventually leads to use of the limited phosphorus pool so that ADP becomes ATP. The extracellular phosphorus then moves to the cells, producing profound hypophosphatemia. This can produce muscular dysfunction, hemolysis, and cardiopulmonary disorders, and may even lead to death (Weisnier and Krumdieck 1981).

2. Kwashiorkor
   a. Occurs rapidly, within 1 to 3 weeks.
   b. Mostly involves decrease of the much smaller pool of the visceral (circulating) proteins. Because this pool is much smaller than the pool of somatic proteins, this malnutrition occurs much faster than the one encountered in marasmus (cachexia).

3. As shown in the table below, visceral proteins are consumed predominantly when there is appreciable glucose and insulin. This is often the case when patients are provided D_5W solution for several days, particularly if they are acutely stressed (Weisnier, Heimburger, and Butterworth 1989). In such a case, the limited calories do not suffice, so breakdown of protein is required. The presence of insulin in hypercatabolic states (as opposed to low insulin in the case of marasmus) protects the protein of muscles and allows the breakdown of the limited pool of visceral protein.

	70 kg		Evaluation		Marasmus (cachexia)	Kwashiorkor
	Man	Woman	Static	Dynamic		
Somatic protein (muscle)	9 kg	7 kg	MAMC† 24-h urea creatinine Bioelectric impedance	N_2 balance	↓	—
Visceral (splachnic) protein (circulating protein)	0.5 kg	0.5 kg	Albumin, transferrin (TIBC), prealbumin	—	—	↓
CHO → CO_2, H_2O, ADP → ATP	0.5 kg	0.5 kg	O_2 consumption			
				$RQ = \dfrac{O_2 \text{ consumption}}{CO_2 \text{ production}}$		—
Lipids → Fat	12 kg	25 kg	TSF‡ Bioelectric impedance		↓	

AA = amino acids; CHO = carbohydrates; I = insulin. Although not shown, other hormones such as glucagon and catecholamines also influence these processes (mostly act to oppose insulin).

† MAMC = mid-arm muscle circumference.

‡ TSF = triceps skin folds.

4. One liter of D_5W contains 200 cal. Thus, anyone fed exclusively by D_5W for a long period may develop kwashiorkor.
5. Kwashiorkor is particularly significant to the ICU patient for two reasons: 1) it occurs with hypercatabolism (increased catecholamines, glucagon, insulin), such as in sepsis and trauma, conditions commonly associated with ventilated patients; and 2) it leads to decreased lymphocytes and host defenses, thus predisposing to sepsis.

F. Assessment of nutritional status in mechanically ventilated patients

1. Baseline fat and protein stores
   a. Fat stores
      i. Triceps skinfold thickness
      ii. Body mass index (BMI) = weight (kg)/height (m^2)
   b. Muscle mass
      i. Limb circumference
      ii. 24-hour urinary creatinine (mg)
   c. Visceral Proteins

Protein	Half-life
Albumin	18 days
Transferrin	8 days
Thyroxin-binding prealbumin	2 days
Retinol-binding protein	12 hours

2. Resisting energy expenditure (REE)
   a. Rough estimation
      Mild stress: 20–30 kcal/kg/d
      Moderate stress: 30–40 kcal/kg/d
      Severe stress: 40–50 kcal/kg/d
   b. Harris-Benedict equation:
      In men, REE = $66.5 + 13.8W + 5.0H - 6.8A$
      In women, REE = $665.1 + 9.6W + 1.8H - 4.7A$
      where
      W = weight (kg)
      H = height (centimeters)
      A = age (years)
      Values are multiplied by stress factor (1.2–2.0, depending on patient's condition).
   c. Direct measurement
      i. Metabolic cart determines $\dot{V}CO_2$, $\dot{V}O_2$, RQ, $\dot{V}E$
      ii. Roughly REE (kcal/d) = $7 \times \dot{V}O_2$ (mL/min)
3. Nitrogen balance
   a. Nitrogen balance = nitrogen input − nitrogen output − 2
      (−2 represents N_2 lost through skin, feces, sweat, and other excreta in which N_2 content is not routinely measured).
   b. Nitrogen input = $\dfrac{\text{Amino acids or protein in grams per day}}{6.25}$
   c. Nitrogen output = 24-hour excretion or urea nitrogen in urine + other excretions (about 2 g/d) + addition of urea nitrogen to body water (i.e., increment in BUN × weight in kilograms × 0.006)
      Example: A 70-kg patient receives 62.5 g of protein daily, has a 24-hour urea nitrogen of 8 g, and his BUN is increased by 20 mg/dL in 24 hours.
      Thus,

$$N_2 \text{ intake} = \frac{62.5}{6.25} = 10 \text{ g/d}$$

and

$$N_2 \text{ output} = 8 \text{ g urine (environment)} + 2 \text{ g (insensible losses)} + 8.4 \text{ g}$$
$$\text{(added to self)} = 18.4 \text{ g}$$

Thus,

$$N_2 \text{ balance} = 10 - 18.4 = 8.4 \text{ g (i.e., he is severely catabolic)}$$

G. Principles of nutritional therapy

1. Carbohydrate and lipids

   a. Needed to replete the energy stores for both immediate use (ATP, creatinine phosphate) and long-term stores (glycogen, fat).

   b. Influence the levels of insulin and other hormones favorably so as to ensure net protein retention (anabolism).

   c. Metabolism

      i. Glucose → One CO_2 produced per one oxygen consumed. Thus, RQ = 1 (RQ = CO_2 production/oxygen consumption).

         a) However, if glucose is used when caloric needs have already been saturated, then glucose + O_2 → fat + 8.7 CO_2. Thus, when glucose is used for lipogenesis, the RQ increases dramatically to 8.7. This is the reason that excessive overfeeding with carbohydrates results in tremendous CO_2 production and respiratory difficulty.

         b) Lipids → RQ = 0.7 (thus, lipids will produce CO_2 at a rate of 30% < glucose)

         c) Thus, in most usual regimens, glucose (or carbohydrates) represents two thirds of calories and lipids represents the remaining one third for a final RQ of 0.9, or about 10% less than if carbohydrates alone were used.

      ii. Overfeeding causes

         a) Excess carbohydrates → fat → fatty liver and increased CO_2 production.

         b) Excess lipids → decreased oxygen diffusion, hyperlipemia, pancreatitis, and infections

      iii. Provide excessive calories only in hypercatabolic states (be suspicious of calories in excess of 40 kcal/kg/day). Be careful because as energy and thus carbohydrates increase, the RQ increases dramatically to 8.7, thus increasing CO_2 production → increased $\dot{V}E$ → increased work of breathing (see Figure 42).

Figure 47

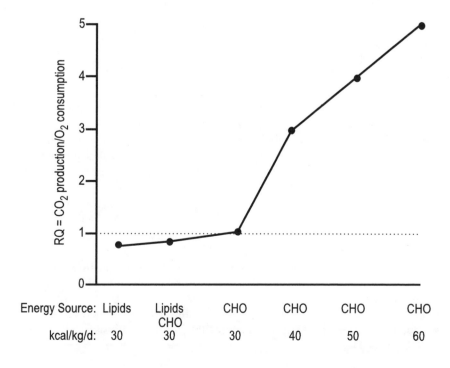

Energy Source:	Lipids	Lipids CHO	CHO	CHO	CHO	CHO
kcal/kg/d:	30	30	30	40	50	60

2. Energy stores: advantages/disadvantages

Carbohydrates		Lipids	
Advantages	Disadvantages	Advantages	Disadvantages
Restoration of ATP (glycolysis) Restoration of glycogen (glycogenesis) Anabolism	$\uparrow CO_2$ production (particularly if energy repletion is excessive) Fatty liver (with excessive calories)	$\downarrow CO_2$ production Good source of energy	$\downarrow O_2$ diffusion (hypoxemia) Immune function impairment Hypertriglyceridemia (uncommon) Pancreatitis (rare)

3. Protein
   a. Necessary to replete protein losses of either muscular origin (somatic protein) or circulating protein (albumin, transferrin, immunoglobulin—splanchnic or visceral proteins).
   b. Most important constituent of formulations.
   c. The decrease in somatic proteins leads to respiratory muscle weakness or may increase the fatigability of the respiratory muscles, which may make patients unable to be weaned from ventilatory support. The decrease in protein does not increase the load to the respiratory system.
   d. Decrease in visceral proteins leads to decreased lymphocytic function and immunoglobulin levels, which in turn lead to infection.
   e. Lowering albumin may lead to poor wound repair.
   f. Overfeeding causes:
      i. Excessive protein (1 g/kg/d or a protein to calorie ratio of >1:30) → excessive urea production → ↑ BUN and ↑ of small nitrogenous waste products → ↓ leucocytic phagocytosis, ↓ platelet adhesiveness, nausea, vomiting, loss of taste, GI bleeding
      ii. Urea → osmotic diuresis → kaliuresis, hypokalemia, hypomagnesemia, arrhythmia, and possibly death
   g. Follow nitrogen kinetics closely and show convincingly that the initial negative nitrogen balance is improving on such a regimen.
4. Calories
   a. Intake should be increased to >30 kcal/kg/d when an extremely catabolic situation is encountered with extremely increased energetic needs, as may be shown directly by ↑ oxygen consumption.

H. **Selection of nutritional prescription**
   1. If use of ventilator is temporary (<3 days), such as in selected cases of respiratory difficulties (overdose, asthma), then no specific nutritional regimen is required.
   2. For expected prolonged ventilatory support (>3 days), nutritional therapy should be started as early as possible.
   3. Route of feeding
      a. Oral route is preferable if patient is able to eat.
      b. Gastric feeding (enteral tube) is preferable if the patient has a good gag reflex and is able to sit in bed.
      c. Duodenal feeding (enteral tube) is preferable for patients who are comatose, who lack a good gag reflex, or who need to be maintained in a horizontal position.
      d. Parenteral feeding is useful if the GI tract cannot be used. Peripheral cannula or central venous line may be used.
   4. Start with:
      • Protein: 1 g/kg/d
      • Carbohydrates: 5 g/kg/d (approximately 20 kcal/kg/d)
      • Lipids: 1 g/kg/d (approximately 10 kcal/kg/d)
      a. In terms of practicality for prescribing central parenteral nutrition:
         • Protein (amino acid solution 10%), approximately 10 mL/kg/d; an average of 600–700 mL/d
         • Lipids 500 mL of 20% solution, approximately 100 g/d ≈ 900 kcal/d
         • Glucose (carbohydrate) approximately 300 g/d ≈ 1200 kcal/d. This is approximately 600 mL of $D_{50}W$

b. Note that lipids are necessary to provide linolenic acid, an essential fatty acid. They do not need to be given daily. However, given the fact that regimens devoid of lipids have significantly more metabolic complications (hypophosphatemia, which could lead to muscular and respiratory difficulties, hypercapnia, fatty liver), daily lipids are given regularly in most ICUs in the United States.

c. Be aware that the formulation indicated above is the one most commonly used. Note that occasionally other formulations to deal with specific diseases may need to be used. For instance, in the case of acute renal failure, the amount of protein may need to be decreased. Similarly, in the case of hepatic failure or major trauma or both, one may elect specific protein formulae that contain higher levels of branched amino acids. In the same vein, one has to be careful when dealing with respiratory disorders; as already mentioned, the total calories and their breakdown (carbohydrates vs. lipids) are extremely important to avoid worsening respiratory insufficiency and difficulty in weaning the patient from the respirator.

d. The nutritional supports used in protein malnutrition syndromes and/or in specific diseases are shown in the tables below.

Nutritional Support in Protein Malnutrition

| Disease | Problems | | |
	Regimen	Underfeeding	Overfeeding
Marasmus (cachexia)	Standard	Minimal, slow repletion	Hypophospholipidemia Heart failure
Kwashiorkor	BCAA*-rich regimen; may consider higher protein and calories than usual (see text)	Inadequate Sepsis ↓ wound healing	Respiratory failure (excessive CO_2 production)

* Branched chain amino acids (leucine, isoleucine, valine).

Nutritional Requirements

Disease	Calories/d	Protein/d
Trauma/sepsis	As many as needed (1.2–1.8 × REE) May use O_2 consumption to indicate needs (see below)	? BCAA-rich* Often 1.2–2 g/kg Use may be determined by N_2 balance
Burns	O_2 consumption REE × 2 for burn area >40% 25 kcal/kg + (40 kcal × % burn area) for burn area <40%	BCAA-rich Note, N_2 output = [urine urea N + (↑ BUN/day × body weight × 60) + (0.2 g × % third-degree burns) + (0.1 g × % second-degree burns) + 4]
Liver disease	30–35 kcal/d	0.6 g/kg "dry" weight
Hepatic encephalopathy	30–35 kcal/d	BCAA-rich Even high amounts acceptable (Cerra et al 1985)
Renal failure		
Acute	30–35 kcal/d	Monitor N_2 balance as needed Specific formula often no advantage (Mirtaldo et al 1982)
Chronic	30–35 kcal/d	0.8 g/kg: no specific formula
Dialysis	30–35 kcal/d	1 g/kg (hemodialysis) 1.2 g/kg (peritoneal dialysis) 1.5 g/kg (peritonitis)
Respiratory failure	30–35 kcal/d	1 g/kg
Cancer	30–35 kcal/d	1 g/kg

* Branched-chain amino acids (leucine, isoleucine, valine).

e. Special care should be taken to ensure appropriate addition of electrolytes/vitamins to maintain stable electrolytic profile.

f. In excessive catabolic states (negative N_2 balance) such as peritonitis, burns, or sepsis, increase the amount of protein or the amount of calories or both. Both maneuvers have been shown to normalize nitrogen balance (see Figure 42). One may need to try to increase protein content or calories (rate of TPN). This should be done while using the N_2 balance to guide the effectiveness of the regimen (with the goal being to achieve an N_2 balance of 0).

Figure 48

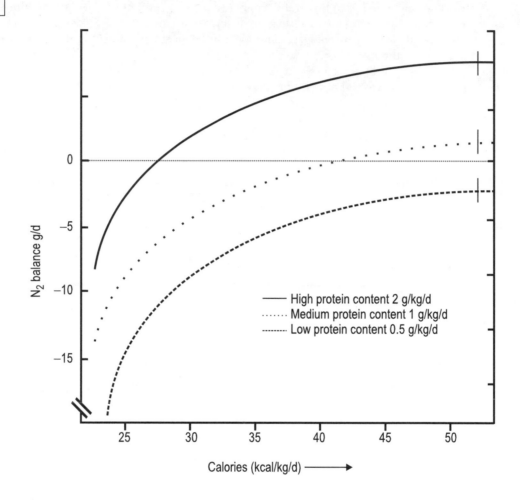

19. Financial Aspects and Prognosis of Patients on Mechanical Ventilation

Suhail Raoof, MD

Naseer Chowdhrey, MD

Faroque A. Khan, MB

> - Use of mechanical ventilation
> - Cost of caring for mechanically ventilated patients
> - Reimbursement practices
> - Cost analysis
> - Methods for curtailing costs

A. Use of mechanical ventilation

1. The use of mechanical ventilation has increased significantly in the last four decades.
2. The reasons for the increased use of mechanical ventilation are multifactorial:
   a. Improved technology for ventilated patients
   b. Ability to keep patients with single or multiple organ failure alive for prolonged periods
   c. Expanded indications for surgery requiring general anesthesia, sedatives, and neuromuscular blocking agents in ICUs
   d. Aging population developing respiratory failure
   e. Patients' heightened expectation of survival during critical illness

B. Cost of caring for mechanically ventilated patients

1. Mechanical ventilation (>2 days) increased daily average hospital costs by 2.36 times the 1975 dollar amount (Davis et al 1980).
2. Average cost of caring for patients mechanically ventilated for ≥2 days was $31,896. (Mayo Clinic Study 1985.)
3. The average duration of hospitalization for mechanically ventilated patients (excluding outliers) was determined to be 41.4 days. The average daily charges for this population of 542 patients in 25 southeastern Wisconsin hospitals was $2285 per day per patient.
4. In a group of 20 mechanically ventilated patients treated at the ICU of Nassau County Medical Center, New York, between July and September 1993, the average costs incurred were as follows:

	n	ICU Total Costs/Patient ($)	ICU Costs/Patient/d ($)	Days in ICU
All Patients	20	9350.95	2286.29	4.098
Major Underlying Diagnosis				
CNS disorder	6	11,145.66	2574.05	4.33
Pulmonary disorder	6	9169.33	2037.63	4.50
Sepsis/ARDS	5	10,865.00	2586.90	4.20
Drug overdose	3	3601.33	1353.88	2.66

Data obtained from Riyaz Bashir, MD, Department of Medicine, Nassau County Medical Center, NY.

5. Wagner determined that the 6% of patients needing mechanical ventilation for >7 days used 37% of the total critical care resources.
6. ICUs siphon off up to 20% of the US health care costs.
7. ICU costs are now approximately 3.0 to 3.8 times greater than those of routine hospital care.

C. Reimbursement practices

1. Health care costs have escalated sevenfold in the United States between 1970 and 1980.
2. Since the introduction of the Diagnosis Related Group (DRG) system, Medicare reimbursement to hospitals is based on the admitting diagnoses of patients. Actual direct costs are not considered for reimbursement purposes.
3. This reimbursement method was found to be grossly inadequate for patients needing prolonged mechanical ventilation.
4. In a group of 95 nonsurgical Medicare patients needing >72 hours of mechanical ventilation (average, 14.2 days), the average loss of revenue to the hospital per discharge was more than $23,000 (1985 US dollars). This study was carried out at Rush–St. Luke's Medical Center in Chicago by Douglass and colleagues (1987).
5. Similar results were found by Gracey and co-workers (1987) in a group of 150 Medicare patients from four hospitals. For those patients who needed >48 hours of mechanical ventilation (average duration, 13 days), hospitals incurred a loss of $20,915 per patient (1985 US dollars).
6. Due to the flaw in the prospective reimbursement pattern of long-term mechanically ventilated patients, the Health Care Financing Administration (HCFA) created two separate DRG categories:
   a. Ventilation through an endotracheal tube (DRG-475), which paid three times more than the average Medicare assignment
   b. Ventilation through a tracheostomy tube (DRG-474), which paid twelve times more than the average Medicare assignment
7. According to the new DRG-483 (patients requiring a tracheostomy for extended mechanical ventilation), reimbursement is still inadequate. Medicare and Medicaid payments for this DRG are approximately 50% and 11% of the charges, respectively.
8. One of the reasons why the new DRG fails to provide adequate compensation is that a primary respiratory diagnosis leading to institution of mechanical ventilation is necessary for increased compensation. This is applicable to only approximately one third of patients.

D. Cost analysis

(Pooled data from Douglass et al [1987], Rosen and Bone [1990], Byrick et al [1980], and Noseworthy et al [1992].)

A breakdown of expenses incurred in caring for mechanically ventilated patients is summarized as follows:

1. Personnel	64%
a. Nursing	44%
b. Respiratory care	20%
2. Investigations	26%
a. Laboratory	20%
b. Radiology	6%
3. Medications (pharmacy)	10%

E. Methods for curtailing costs

1. Minimizing the duration of mechanical ventilation
   a. As many as one third of patients who self-extubate do not need reintubation. This may indicate that patients may not be extubated quickly enough. Additional ventilator days may prolong ICU stay and add to spiraling medical costs.
   b. Kollef and colleagues (1997) studied the duration of mechanical ventilation, using predetermined weaning protocols implemented by nurses and respiratory therapists automatically or by physicians.
      i. After predetermined weaning parameters were fulfilled, patients were weaned using spontaneous breathing trials, pressure support, or intermittent mandatory ventilation. The results are summarized as follows:

	n	Total Duration of Ventilation (h)	Reintubation (%)
Physician directed	178	102.0 ± 169.1	23.6
Protocol directed	179	69.4 ± 123.7	22.3

    ii. Shorter duration of mechanical ventilation translated into reduced patient discomfort and a savings of $42,960 in hospital costs over 4 months in their centers.

  c. To shorten the duration of mechanical ventilation, we implement the following weaning guidelines in most patients:

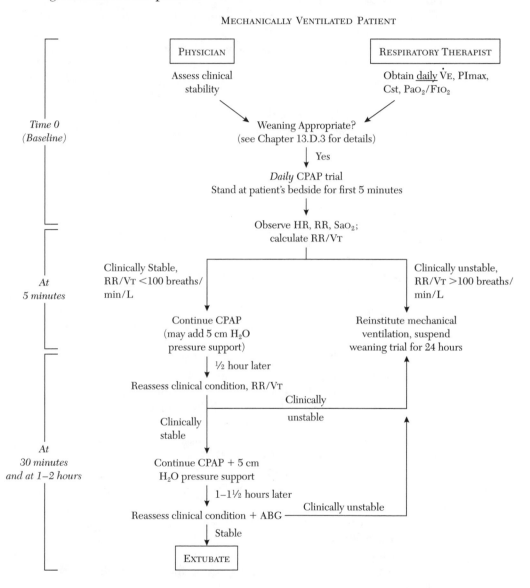

MECHANICALLY VENTILATED PATIENT

2. Conserving existing resources

  a. Arterial blood gases

    i. ABGs in ventilated patients may be unnecessary in up to 50% of cases (Civetta and Hudson-Civetta 1985).

    ii. Checking ABGs account for most laboratory expenses.

    iii. Such reductions may translate into significant cost savings.

    iv. Pulse oximetry may be a useful alternative in many patients.

v. ABGs do not necessarily need to be checked at every ventilator setting change in patients who are being weaned.

b. Ventilator circuit

    i. In the past, ventilator circuits were changed every 24 hours.

    ii. The incidence of nosocomial pneumonia did not increase when the frequency of ventilator change was reduced from 24 hours to 48 hours.

    iii. Dreyfuss and colleagues (1991) demonstrated that the incidence of pneumonia was 31% when ventilator circuits were changed every 24 hours compared with 29% when they were never changed for the entire duration of mechanical ventilation.

    iv. The Centers for Disease Control recommends that the practice of daily change in ventilator circuits may be extended to >48 hours.

    v. In our hospital, a circuit change costs $14. By reducing the incidence of ventilator circuit change from 1 day to 7 days, the hospital saved over $92,000 per year (excluding the time it takes for the respiratory therapist to change circuits).

c. Daily CXR examinations

    i. Portable CXRs may constitute as many as 40%–50% of all chest examinations.

    ii. Occasionally, portable films are suboptimal owing to inability to capture detail and full information, and inability to regulate accurately the exposure of the film.

    iii. In a review of three radiology studies, routine daily CXRs showed unexpected findings in only 37%, 43%, and 55% of cases.

    iv. Appropriate indications to perform portable CXRs on mechanically ventilated patients generally include:

        a) Confirmation of clinical suspicion of pneumonia

        b) Heart failure

        c) Atelectasis

        d) Barotrauma

        e) Device or apparatus position or placement

        f) Mediastinal problems or pulmonary hemorrhage

    v. Routine daily CXRs in mechanically ventilated patients should be discouraged.

d. Use of metered-dose inhalers (instead of nebulizers)

    i. β-agonists administered by metered-dose inhalers are as effective as when administered by nebulizers.

    ii. Metered-dose inhaler substitutions are possible in >60% of nebulized aerosol treatments.

       • Bowton and colleagues (1992) showed that three puffs from a metered-dose inhaler placed in the inspiratory limb of the ventilator circuit reduced the cost of delivery to $5 compared with $13 for a single nebulized treatment (cost savings of approximately $83,000 annually in their hospital).

3. Prevention of complications of mechanical ventilation

a. Utilize lung protection strategies such as permissive hypercapnia, pressure-targeted ventilation, and Pel measurements (Section III.15.C)

b. Avoid oxygen toxicity (Section III.15.F on oxygen toxicity)

c. Minimize risks of nosocomial pneumonia and atelectasis (see section III.15.D on complications of mechanical ventilation)

    i. Elevation of head of bed by at least 30 degrees

    ii. Continuous suctioning of subglottic secretions

    iii. Minimizing gastric residue with tube feeding

    iv. Continuous postural oscillations ± percussion therapy in high-risk patients

4. Rationing hospital resources

a. Discussion of Advance Directives:

    i. The patient should decide if he or she wants the quality of life that mechanical ventilation offers; however this decision should be made *before* mechanical ventilation is used.

    ii. Patients with severe chronic obstructive pulmonary disease, progressive neuromuscular disorders, AIDS, and terminal cancers should be informed of the possibility of remaining intubated and mechanically ventilated long term.

iii. Long-term mechanical ventilation of chronically debilitated individuals may turn out to be a financially draining proposition, both for the patient and the hospital.

iv. In a group of 50 amyotrophic lateral sclerosis patients who consented for an interview, 38 (76%) had completed Advance Directives. Seventy-six percent of patients wanted long-term mechanical ventilation to be discontinued in specific situations.

b. Application of outcome-based studies to decide who should have mechanical ventilation

i. Examine the likelihood of survival when mechanical ventilation is used, based on the specific disease. Patients projected to have a very poor prognosis may not be considered candidates for mechanical ventilation.

ii. Some studies of patients who were mechanically ventilated are summarized as follows:

Disease	Study Period	Mortality	Author
AIDS with *Pneumocystis* pneumonia	1981–1985	86%	Wachter et al (1995)
	1986–1988	61%	
	1989–1991	76%	
ARDS	1993	10%–90%*	Bernard et al (1994)
COPD (>48 h ventilatory support)	1988	34%	Swinburne et al (1988)
Cardiac arrest	1990	80%	Rosen and Bone (1990)
Malignancy	1988	92%	Peters et al (1988)

* Wide variation, depending on the cause of ARDS.

iii. Comparative risk of dying of acute respiratory failure, according to specific disease categories, in a group of 383 mechanically ventilated patients (Stauffer et al 1993)
   a) Postoperative respiratory failure   0.93
   b) Chronic obstructive pulmonary disease (COPD)   1.00
   c) Pneumonia   1.09
   d) Cardiogenic pulmonary edema   1.69
   e) Cardiac or respiratory arrest   2.88

iv. In mechanically ventilated patients with COPD, Menzies and colleagues (1989) found that survival was best determined by:
   a) Activity level prior to institution of mechanical ventilation
   b) Level of dyspnea (ATS score)
   c) FEV_1 (>40% → 60% survived)
   d) Serum albumin levels

v. In a study by Rieves et al (1993) the factor most strongly associated with poor prognosis in patients with severe COPD was the presence of CXR infiltrates at the time of intubation:

CXR Infiltrates*

	Survivors	Non-survivors	P Value
FEV_1 <1L	9.1%	94.2%	0.001
FEV_1 >1L	54.5%	87.5%	0.127

* Mainly bacterial pneumonias, congestive heart failure.

Thus, patients with severe chronic obstructive pulmonary disease and pulmonary infiltrates had the worst prognosis.

vi. Other variables predicting poor prognosis are:
   a) Age >70 years
   b) Serum albumin <20 g/L
   c) APACHE II score >35[†]
   d) Cardiopulmonary resuscitation leading to mechanical ventilation (Papadakis et al 1993)

[†] Mortality on Day 4 of patients with medical and surgical problems, excluding myocardial infarctions, coronary artery bypass grafting any operation, and burns were as follows: APACHE II score 0–10: up to 30%; score 11–20: up to 60%; score 21–25: up to 73% (score >25: up to 97%) (Knaus 1989).

vii. Most studies show that duration of mechanical ventilation does not correlate with prognosis.
viii. Decisions to provide mechanical ventilation based on cost-benefit-outcome data may become difficult to uphold.
ix. Severity of both the acute and chronic medical illness, patient age, and functional states may be taken into consideration in the APACHE scores or other similar prognostication systems.
x. Ethically a mortality figure derived from a group of patients may not be applicable to an individual patient.
xi. Economic constraints should not be considered an overriding factor in the decision to provide mechanical ventilation.

5. Creation of step-down respiratory care units in hospitals
   a. With the refinement of noninvasive monitoring techniques (especially pulse oximetry and end-tidal CO_2 monitoring), technologically improved mechanical ventilators, and the understanding that weaning may take several weeks in some patients, step-down respiratory care units were cautiously created and tested.
   b. By reducing the nurse:patient ratio, excluding invasive monitoring, developing simple treatment protocols, and utilizing case managers to care for hemodynamically stable patients, significant cost savings may accrue.
   c. The results of outcomes of some of these step-down units are summarized in the table below:

Author	Year/Duration of Study	Respiratory Unit Description	Monitoring	Duration of Stay (days)	Advantages
Krieger et al (1994)	1988 (2 y)	Central station non-invasive monitoring N:P::1:5–6	R + C	26	• Cost of care $328 less than ICU • Cost savings/y $140,063
Raoof et al (1991)	1991 (1 y)	14 separate rooms Audible ventilator disconnect alarms N:P::1:4 One dedicated respiratory therapist	R (−) C (−)	85	• Weaning success 54% • Average boarding cost per patient weaned: $12,350 (vs. $25,440 in MICU)
Elpern et al (1990)	1990 (1 y)	Noninvasive respiratory care unit—11 beds Private medical floor beds with rail system, surveillance cameras N:P::1:3–5	R + C	16.2 days for 78% patients	• Cost savings of $1976 per patient per day as compared to MICU • Cost of care was reduced by $20,000 per patient
Scheinhorn et al (1994)	1994 (3 y)	Regional weaning center (RWC)—49 beds Located within general care areas Run by case management teams using critical pathways N:P::1:4–5 (ICU 1:1–1:2)	R (+) C (+)	39 (46.9 ± 2.9 for patients successfully weaned)	• 53% weaning success • 71% survived to discharge • Cost reduction per patient per day between ICU and RWC is $1500 • Approximately $208 per patient per day less costly than noninvasive respiratory care unit
Latriano (1996)	1996 (4.5 y)	9-bed nonmonitored respiratory care floor Part of a 20-bed general medical floor Tracheostomy preferred N:P::1:3 (Medical floor 1:7)	R (−) C (−)	49	• 50% patients survived (APACHE score of 16.5) • 90% survivors intubated • 6% of survivors needed long-term ventilator facility • Cost of care $453 per patient per day (ICU: $830 per patient per day)

R = respiratory monitoring; C = cardiac monitoring.
* Average duration of stay.

6. Transferring patients to long-term facilities (nursing homes capable of caring for mechanically ventilated patients)
   a. Costs
      i. The costs incurred would depend on:
         a) Personnel caring for the patient
         b) Type of ventilator and equipment used
         c) Level of care that the patient's condition warrants
         d) Local factors.
      ii. Projected costs of caring for mechanically ventilated patients are approximately one fourth to one tenth those of an acute care center (hospital).
      iii. In a survey of long-term ventilatory support in Minnesota carried out by Adams and colleagues in 1986, the entire monthly costs in a long-term care facility were $19,351 (in contrast to patients in MICU where monthly expenses were $64,513).
   b. Proposed criteria to be fulfilled for transfer from a hospital to a chronic care facility:
      i. Clinical
         a) Nonpulmonary
            • Patient must be clinically and hemodynamically stable (no life-threatening arrhythmias).
            • No major testing or change in treatment regimen is expected for at least 1 month.
            • Nutritional support has been instituted and optimized for several days.
         b) Pulmonary
            • Need for long-term mechanical ventilation is firmly established (underlying cause of respiratory failure is not likely to reverse), and patient has failed weaning attempts.
            • Stable respiratory status (no pneumonia, atelectasis, etc.).
            • Absence of dyspnea.
            • Acceptable ABGs without need for PEEP, high $\dot{V}E$ or $FIO_2 > 0.40$ for ≥ 24 hours.
            • Absence of copious secretions (that need frequent suctioning).
            • Tracheostomy tube has been placed ≥ 24 hours earlier.
            • Methods of communication have been tried and tested with patient, if applicable.
      ii. Nonclinical
         a) Patient and/or family consents to transfer.
         b) Patient is psychologically prepared to go to chronic care facility, if alert and oriented.
         c) Chronic care facility accepts patient.
         d) The patient and/or family has been taught some basic and essential aspects of the ventilator management, suctioning, care of tracheostomy site, etc.
   c. Experience of caring for mechanically ventilated patients at A. Holly Patterson Geriatric Center (AHPNH) (affiliated with Nassau County Medical Center)
      N. Chowdhrey, MD; S. Raoof, MD; C. Carvounis, MD; P. Scrak, BBA; R. Gumpeni, MD; F. Khan, MB
      i. Beds
         a) General: 900
         b) Mechanically ventilated: 30
      ii. Occupancy rate of ventilated beds: almost always 100%

iii. Staffing
   a) One pulmonologist (one-half day) covers approximately 80 patients, including ventilated patients (provides coverage for 4 hours on Saturday and Sunday). Night and weekend coverage by internist on call.

Shifts	Respiratory Therapist	Nurses	Nurses' Aide
7 a.m.–3 p.m.	6*	4	3
3 p.m.–11 p.m.	3	3	4
11 p.m.–7 a.m.	2	3	3–4

   * For entire nursing home. Approximately 80% of the respiratory therapist's time is spent in the ventilator ward.

iv. Ventilators used: Puritan–Bennett 2800
v. Personnel responsibilities
   a) Physicians
      • Brief weekly examination
      • Detailed monthly evaluation
      • Sick sites visits as needed
      • Monthly multidisciplinary care planning meetings
   b) Respiratory therapist
      • Daily rounds on patients and ventilator checks
      • Suction respiratory secretions p.r.n.
      • ABGs (on admission and p.r.n.)
      • Change ventilator tubing once per month
      • Heat moisture exchanger (humidifier) change every 24 hours and p.r.n.
      • Change tracheostomy tube every 6 weeks
      • Help in giving showers to patients once per week and take them outside the ventilator ward
   c) Nursing
      • Usual nursing responsibilities (dispensing medications, checking vital signs every shift, direct patient care).
      • Reposition patient p.r.n.
      • Check for alarms, equipment malfunctions, or disconnections from ventilators. Observe ventilated patients a minimum of every 30 min.
      • Give nasogastric feeding every shift.
      • Change tracheostomy tube; provide tracheostomy care and suctioning.
      • Give showers to patients once per week.
vi. Patient demographics and survival
   • (n = 60 patients)
   • Study period = 3 years
   • Sex distribution: 39 females, 21 males

Age Range (years)	Females	Males	Survivors	Nonsurvivors
<50	4	2	1	5
50–65	6	9	5	10
65–75	8	3	6	5
<75	21	7	9	19
Percentage	—	—	35%	65%
Diagnosis*				
COPD	16	10	7	19
Neurologic disorders	18	11	12	17

   * The remainder of the cases belong to miscellaneous diagnoses. Only the two major diagnoses that account for >90% of the cases are shown.

Survival Graph for Nursing Home Residents

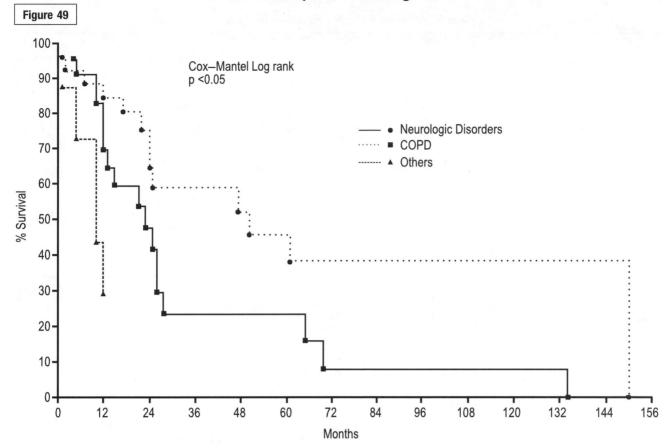

Neurologic diseases and COPD accounted for >90% of cases studied. Hazard function analysis demonstrated that the expected mean survival of patients with neurologic diseases is 72.13 months whereas that of COPD patients is 33.22 months.

vii. Causes of death ($n = 39$)

Reason	n	Total (%)
Pneumonia	16	41
Acute respiratory failure	4	10
Sepsis	6	15
Cardiac causes (MI, CHF, arrhythmias)	5	13
Acute renal failure	4	10
Gastrointestinal bleeding	1	3
Anoxic brain damage	3	8

viii. General reimbursement policy at AHPNH

Mechanically Ventilated Patients Reimbursement/Patient/Day ($)

Year	Days	Medicare	Medicaid	Patient Co-Payment
1987*	1–20	$80.30	—	—
	21–100	$15.30	—	$65.00
	>100	None[†]	$118.83[‡]	—
1989*	1–8	$64.50	—	$25.50
	9–150	$90.00	—	—
	>150	—	$144.66[‡]	—
1990		Same as 1987; Act of 1989 was repealed		
1992[§]	1–20	$90.00	$363.33	—
(Nov 25)	21–100	$8.50	$363.33	$81.50
	>100	—	$363.33	—
1996[‖]	All days	$413.82[¶] or $288.24	—	—

*After 3-day minimum hospital stay.

[†]With minor exceptions, there was a ceiling of 100 days for reimbursement in the lifetime of a patient receiving nursing care.

[‡]For skilled nursing care once eligibility criteria are met.

[§]The nursing home received approval for a distinct Medicaid reimbursement rate for mechanically ventilated patients.

[‖] Medicare developed a case mix demonstration project in which additional reimbursement rate was established depending on complexity of illness.

[¶] Reimbursement according to ADL score (takes into consideration eating, feeding, and toilet capabilities of patient).

Specific expenses versus reimbursement rate (for 1996):
   a) Actual cost of caring for patients on mechanical ventilation (e.g., personnel, pharmacy, labs and investigations, ECG, diet) was $495.50/day
      • Drug costs were $12.00/day.
   b) Total cost of operating a 20-bed ventilator unit was $3,600,000/year or $180,000/bed/year.
   c) Medicaid reimbursement rate was $432.87/day.
      • Average loss of revenue per patient per day was $62.63 (in contrast to a loss of $1,538.18 per day per patient if such patients were kept in the medical ICU on a long-term basis).
      • Average yearly loss of revenue per patient per year $22,860.
   d) Losses incurred per year in caring for 20 mechanically ventilated patients at AHPNH were $457,200 (assuming a 100% census of the 20 beds).
7. Home care for long-term mechanically ventilated patients
   a. Less expensive than even chronic care facilities.
   b. Adams and colleagues (1993) determined the average cost of ventilatory support at home to be $6557 per month compared with $19,557 per month in a chronic care facility.
   c. Cost of caring for patients at home may also depend on who is allowed to care for, and suction from, tracheostomies. If state laws mandate licensed nurses and not other home attendants, the cost of home care increases significantly.
   d. Special considerations in providing ventilatory support at home
      i. General
         a) Patient wants to return home.
         b) Family members want the patient at home.
         c) A support system exists within the family to help with the patient's care (in most instances).
         d) Patient's condition is stable.
         e) It has been determined that the patient will need life-long ventilatory support.
         f) The patient, if possible, and family have been taught aspects of ventilatory care, including suctioning and tracheostomy care.

ii. Ventilator related
 a) Positive-pressure ventilation (pressure targeted; volume targeted)
  - Noninvasive (e.g., BiPAP)
    Continuous
    Intermittent (e.g., nocturnal ventilation)
  - Invasive
    Continuous
    Intermittent
 b) Negative-pressure ventilation
  - Cuirass
  - Pulmowrap
  - Body tank
 c) Modes of ventilation (see Section II.4.G)
 d) Power supply
  - Electronic
  - Battery (e.g., car battery)
    For mobility
    For frequent power failures
    As a back-up
 e) Mobility
  - Transported on wheelchair
  - Transported on a pole
  - Nonportable (i.e., stays in room)
 f) Oxygen supply
  - To maintain PaO_2 ≥60 mm Hg or SaO_2 ≥90%
  - Methods for providing oxygen
    Gas tanks containing oxygen
    Oxygen concentrator
    Liquid oxygen tanks
 g) Maintenance issues
  - Ventilator circuits
  - Humidification
  - Endotracheal tubes/mask
  - Ventilator checks
iii. Patient–ventilator interface (for positive-pressure ventilation)
 a) Tracheostomy tube
  - Plastic or metal
  - Cuffed or uncuffed
  - Fenestrated or nonfenestrated
 b) Mouthpiece
 c) Face mask
  - Nasal mask
  - Full-face mask
iv. Respiratory secretion suctioning equipment
v. Patient communication issues
 a) Face mask vs. tracheostomy tubes
 b) Deflation of cuff of tracheostomy tube
 c) Cuffed tracheostomy tubes with an attached narrow diameter tube with its distal opening near proximal end of cuff (e.g., Portex cuffed tracheostomy speaking tube, Portex, Inc., Nashua, NH; Pitt cuffed tracheostomy speaking tube, Mallinckrodt Critical Care, St. Louis, MO)
 d) Uncuffed tubes or fenestrated tubes
 e) Special unidirectional valves to facilitate speaking, (e.g., *Passy-Muir tracheostomy speaking valves*, Passy & Muir, Irvine, CA; *Kristner Valve*, Pilling Rusch Corp, Fort Washington, PA; *Olympic Valve*, Olympic Medical Corp., Seattle, WA; *Montgomery Valve*, Boston Medical Products, Waltham, MA)

IV. APPENDIX

1. Basics of Ventilatory Support

Faroque A. Khan, MB

Suhail Raoof, MD

A. Practical guidelines for assessment of need for mechanical ventilation

Process	Usual Indication(s)	Useful Parameters	Comments
Acute respiratory failure without underlying chronic respiratory disease			
a. Neuromuscular illness (e.g., Guillain–Barré syndrome, myasthenia gravis, stroke, drug overdose)	Imminent failure of respiratory pump; recurrent atelectasis, unstable respiratory drive; absent gag reflex; ICP needs to be lowered	Maximum inspiratory pressure <25 cm H_2O; vital capacity <15 mL/kg; RR >35–40/min	Onset of abnormalities in gas exchange is often sudden and occurs after signs of weakness.
b. Central airway obstruction (e.g., central airway tumors, vocal cord dysfunction)	Presence of inspiratory stridor; central cyanosis	Rising $PaCO_2$	Emergency tracheostomy may be necessary.
c. Lung parenchymal or airway disease (e.g., ARDS, pulmonary edema, pneumonia, asthma)	Progressive refractory hypoxemia; progressive respiratory acidosis; excessive work of breathing; decreased consciousness; exhaustion	PaO_2 <60 mm Hg, with FIO_2 >0.6; $PaCO_2$ increases 5–10 mm Hg above baseline; pH <7.3; RR >35–40/min	Hypercapnia is often a late manifestation, especially in asthma.
d. Circulatory failure (e.g., myocardial infarction, cardiogenic shock)	Refractory hypotension; increased oxygen consumption; increased $PaCO_2$	As above for lung parenchymal disease (c) (up to 50% cardiac output may be diverted to respiratory muscles)	The failing or ischemic myocardium has to cope with the additional work that the exercising respiratory muscles demand.
e. Stupor or coma (e.g., drug overdose)	Airway protection	Poor gag reflex, ineffective cough	Onset of apnea may be abrupt.
Acute-on-chronic respiratory failure (e.g., acute exacerbations of COPD or chronic neuromuscular disease)	Impaired mental status, refractory hypoxemia; progressive respiratory acidosis	PaO_2 <35–40 mm Hg despite controlled oxygen therapy; pH <7.20–7.25; RR >35–40/min	Implies hypoxemia or CO_2 narcosis; oxygen therapy resulting in progressive respiratory acidosis is an indication for mechanical ventilation.

B. Clinical guidelines for mechanical ventilation in specific conditions
(Includes recommendations from the ACCP consensus conference on mechanical ventilation)
1. ARDS
   a. Mode of ventilation: Initially assisted mode is commonly used. If conventional ventilation fails, consider pressure controlled ± inverse ratio or high-frequency positive-

pressure ventilation with extracorporeal CO_2 removal (there is no definite proof that one mode is better than the other).

b. Start with VT 10 mL/kg. Lower to as low as 5–7 mL/kg within 24–48 hours, if possible.

c. Keep FIO_2 ≤0.6, if possible, to keep PaO_2 at 55–57 mm Hg. (It is acceptable to keep SaO_2 slightly <90%.)

d. Use PEEP (determine optimal PEEP daily) to improve oxygenation, minimizing FIO_2. PEEP may be set 1–2 cm above lower inflection point.

e. Monitor Pel with an aim to keep it ≤35 cm H_2O.

f. Allow $PaCO_2$ to increase (permissive hypercapnia) to allow lowering of Pel to ≤35 cm H_2O if necessary. This strategy can be deployed in the setting of ARDS unless the patient has a risk factor for increased intracranial tension or has serious arrhythmias or hypotension.

g. If acceptable levels of oxygenation are not achieved, consider sedation ± paralysis, improvement of oxygen delivery (increasing cardiac output and hemoglobin), prone position ventilation, use of intravenous oxygenation system, or high-frequency ventilation. (High-frequency oscillation is not currently FDA-approved for adults.)

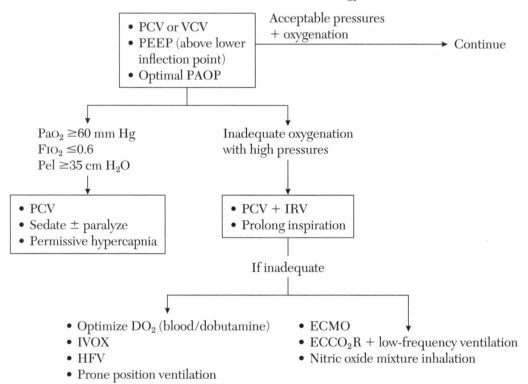

Severe ARDS
Mechanical Ventilation Strategy

2. Obstructive airways disease (asthma/COPD)

a. Mode of ventilation initially is volume- or pressure-targeted and usually assisted. (The institution of assisted ventilation [volume cycled] in the awake or agitated patient may be associated with hyperinflation from air trapping. Consider alternative modes, such as SIMV after stabilizing the patient.)

b. Use the lowest V̇E that allows an acceptable gas exchange to occur. Permissive hypercapnia is a reasonable option for minimizing dynamic hyperinflation.

c. Increase peak flows (~80 L/min) in VCV to decrease inspiratory time and to allow more time for expiration. (Monitor impact of increasing peak flows on PIP.)

d. In the presence of dynamic hyperinflation, apply small amounts of ventilator-applied PEEP.

e. If the patient is fighting the ventilator, exclude hypoxemia and other treatable conditions. Then consider sedation ± paralysis.

Severe Asthma/COPD

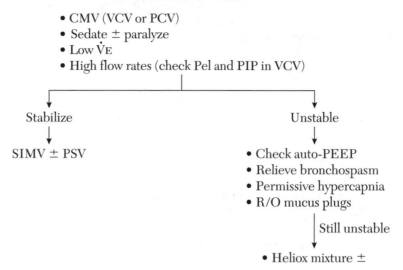

- CMV (VCV or PCV)
- Sedate ± paralyze
- Low $\dot{V}E$
- High flow rates (check Pel and PIP in VCV)

Stabilize

SIMV ± PSV

Unstable

- Check auto-PEEP
- Relieve bronchospasm
- Permissive hypercapnia
- R/O mucus plugs

Still unstable

- Heliox mixture ±

3. Neuromuscular diseases
   a. Assisted mode (volume control) is preferable.
   b. Larger V_T (12–15 mL/kg) to prevent atelectasis and to improve dyspnea is appropriate.
   c. Higher peak inspiratory flow rates (~80 L/min) will help in allaying the dyspnea that these patients have.
   d. Strictly enforcing that Pels be <35 cm H_2O is less important than in ARDS, because patients generally do not have intrinsic restrictive lung disease. Thus, they are at less risk of barotrauma than patients with restrictive lung disease.
   e. Consider pressure support while weaning patients with borderline muscle strength and nocturnal positive pressure, once they are extubated.
4. Head trauma
   a. Maintain eucapnia for patients with stable head injury
   b. Elevated ICP: maintain $PaCO_2$ 25–30 mm Hg
      i. Return $PaCO_2$ to baseline gradually over 24 hours
5. Myocardial ischemia
   a. Choose modes of mechanical ventilation that minimize work of breathing.
   b. Positive-pressure ventilation may have beneficial effects in patients with LVF/CHF by decreasing venous return and decreasing pulmonary vascular congestion (see Case 5, pp 155–156, for further description).
   c. Positive-pressure ventilation, especially with PEEP, may make the hemodynamic data obtained from a right heart catheter less reliable. (See "Monitoring During Mechanical Ventilation," pp 56–68)
6. Postoperative patients
   a. If no underlying lung disease exists, attempt to extubate rapidly past postanesthetic period.
   b. ? ± Pressure Support Ventilation. (It was shown by Prakash and Meij that PSV was well tolerated and weaning time significantly reduced in the postoperative period. Due to better patient acceptance of this mode, the need for heavy sedation and muscular paralysis was minimized.)
7. Bronchopleural fistula
   a. Mode of ventilation: conventional modes such as assist control or SIMV usually suffice.
   b. If the air leak is not large and the patient can be adequately ventilated, the following measures should be taken to expedite healing and thus closure of fistula:
      i. Use lowest V_T to allow acceptable ventilation.

  ii. Permissive hypercapnia is appropriate; if necessary, lower peak and plateau pressures.
  iii. Minimize PEEP, if possible.
  iv. Lower chest tube suction pressures.
 c. If the patient cannot be adequately ventilated (despite high inspiratory flow rates and large V_T), consider independent lung ventilation.

C. Initial ventilator settings

Mode:	Assist/control
V_T:	10–12 mL/kg
Rate (Back-up):	12 breaths/min
F_{IO_2}:	0.40–1.0
Flow rate:	40–80 L/min
PEEP:	None

I:E ratio of 1:3
Pressure alarm: 10 cm H_2O above initial peak pressure

D. Initial ventilator management

1. Check ABG approximately 20 minutes after initiation of mechanical ventilation and every 20–30 minutes thereafter until the patient is stabilized.
2. Adjust F_{IO_2} to maintain PaO_2 between 60 and 100 mm Hg.
3. Adjust $\dot{V}E$ ($V_T \times f$) to achieve a desired $PaCO_2$ that results in a near normal pH (i.e., 7.40). The exception would be when using permissive hypercapnia. Use the equation:

$$\text{Desired } \dot{V}E = \frac{\text{Present } PaCO_2}{\text{Desired } PaCO_2} \times \text{Present } \dot{V}E$$

4. The flow rate and I:E ratio may need to be adjusted and the flow rate may need to be increased in patients with high inspiratory demands (this may decrease work of breathing, improve patient comfort, and decrease auto-PEEP).

E. Criteria suggesting successful weaning

a. Respiratory muscle strength
 i. Maximum inspiratory pressure more negative than -30 cm H_2O
 ii. Maximum voluntary ventilation of greater than two times resting $\dot{V}E$
b. Ventilatory demands
 i. Spontaneous RR <35/min
 ii. Resting $\dot{V}E$ <10 L
 iii. V_D/V_T <0.6
c. Ventilatory mechanics
 i. Vital capacity of >15 mL/kg body weight
 ii. Static compliance >33 mL/cm H_2O
d. Oxygenation
 i. $D(A\text{-}a)O_2$ <350
 ii. $\dfrac{PaO_2}{F_{IO_2}} >200$
 iii. Shunt fraction ($\dot{Q}s/\dot{Q}T$) $<20\%$

2. Diagrammatic Representations

Douglas Colquhoun, RRT

Figure 50

Note: A, B, and E: ventilator breaths; C and D: patient's own breaths; F, G, and J correspond to set V_T; H and I correspond to the patient's V_T

SIMV Ventilation Waveform Patterns

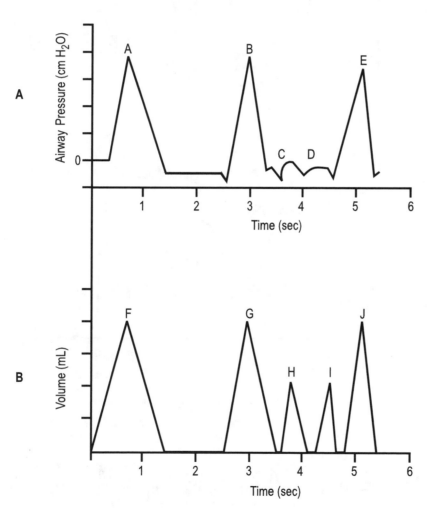

Figure 51

A-B and C-D indicate that flow ceases towards the end of inpiration; however, exhalation does not start immediately. Inspiration holds. A higher VT cannot be obtained at these settings. E-F and G-H indicate that flow does not return to zero and that therefore inspiration could be prolonged to increase VT.

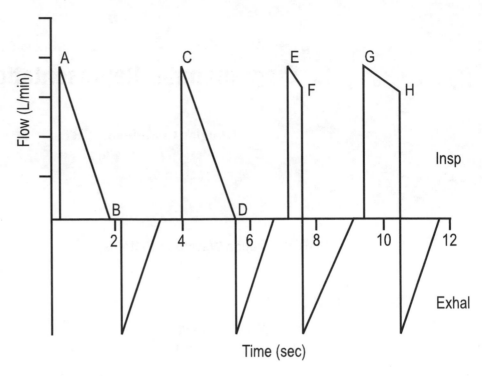

Figure 52

A-B-C represents no patient effort or control ventilation. D-E-F shows a slight decrease in pressure, which indicates that the patient is making an effort to breathe.

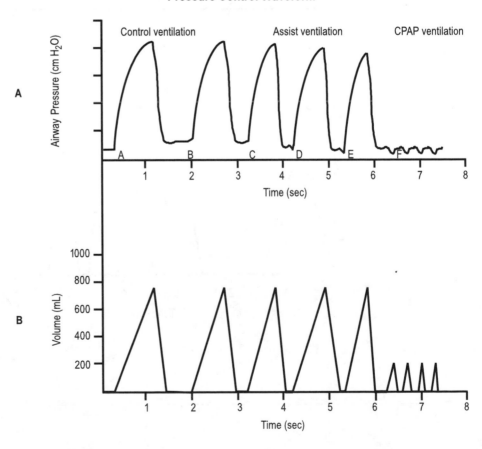

Pressure Control Waveform

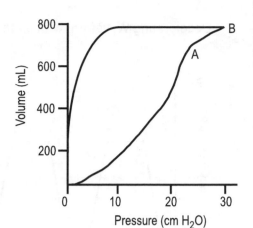

Figure 53

There is little volume increase from A-B but big pressure changes. This is an example of lung over-distention.

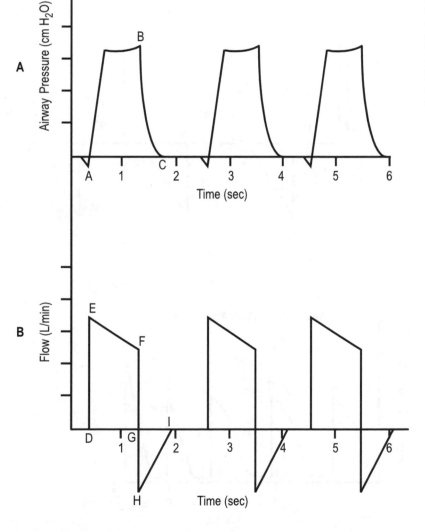

Pressure Support Waveform Patterns

Figure 54

Point A: patient's inspiratory effort. Ventilator then reaches preset pressure support value and maintains that pressure. Ventilator cycles off at point B and returns to baseline at point C. Point D indicates that inspiratory flow starts and reaches a maximum at point E, where flow begins to taper off. Inspiratory flow ends at point F. Points G-H-I: expiratory flow.

Figure 55

Normal waveform pattern. Note:
A-B indicates plateau or hold time;
C-D indicates no inspiratory or
expiratory flow.

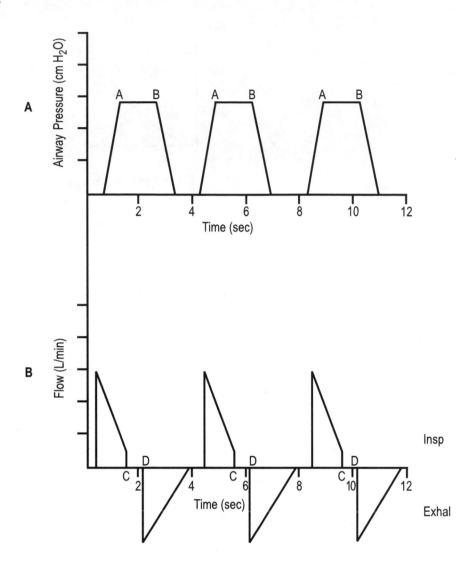

Decelerating Waveform with an Inspiratory Hold Time

Figure 56

A-B-C: If inspiratory flow rate is
too low for the patient, the patient
will work harder to breathe. Point D
indicates no lag in slope or peak
pressure. Flow rate is enough at this
time. Point E indicates an excessive
inspiratory flow rate that may not be
comfortable for the patient. Too
quick a peak inspiratory flow rate
may increase peak inspiratory
pressure too quickly and cause
barotrauma.

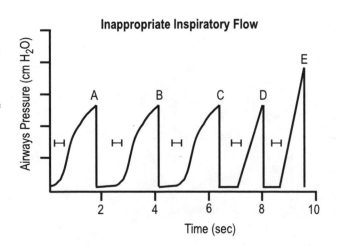

Inappropriate Inspiratory Flow

Efficacy of Bronchodilator Therapy

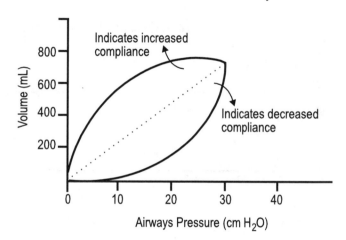

Pressure-Volume Loop

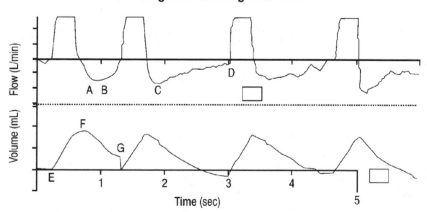

Diagrams Showing Auto-PEEP

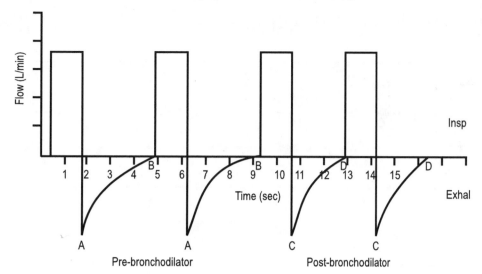

Figure 57

A-B indicates that a longer exhalation time is needed. C-D indicates that a shorter exhalation time is needed.

Figure 58

Figure 59

A-B: incomplete exhalation; C-D: incomplete exhalation; E-F: delivered vital volume; F-G: exhaled vital volume. Note: Exhaled V_T is less than delivered vital volume. Respirator cycled on before exhalation was complete. Air trapping occurred at this point.

Figure 60

A-B: inspiration; B: end of inspiration, beginning of exhalation; B-C-D: expiratory flow. Note: Expiratory flow continues as inspiration starts again at point D. Vᴛ remains constant. Patient has intrinsic PEEP.

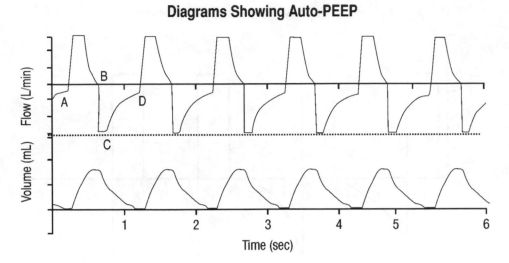

Diagrams Showing Auto-PEEP

Figure 61

Peak pressures on top graph. Inspiratory and expiratory flows on bottom graph. A-B: inspiration; B: peak pressure. C-D: inspiration; D-E-F: expiration.

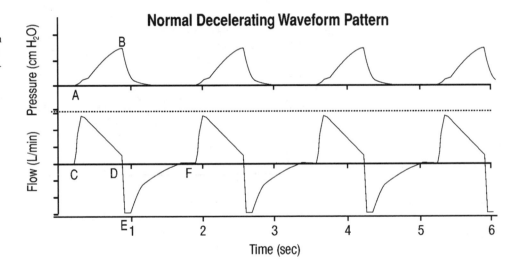

Normal Decelerating Waveform Pattern

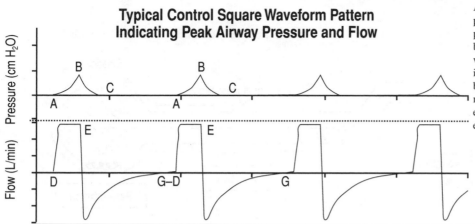

Typical Control Square Waveform Pattern Indicating Peak Airway Pressure and Flow

A: beginning of inspiration (baseline pressure); B: peak inspiratory pressure; C: pressure returns to baseline; D-E: ventilator square wave flow pattern; D: beginning of inspiration; E: end of inspiration, beginning of exhalation; F: maximum expiratory flow; G: end of expiratory flow; G-D: time between exhalation and inhalation.

Figure 62

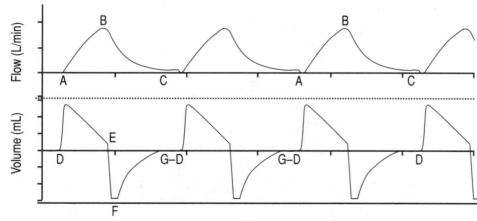

Typical Control Decelerating Waveform Pattern Indicating Flow and Volume

A: beginning of inspiration; B: end of inspiration, beginning of exhalation; C: end of exhalation; D-E: ventilator decelerating flow pattern—inspiration; E: exhalation begins; F: maximum exhalation flow; G: end of expiratory flow; G-D: pause between next break.

Figure 63

Compliance
• Resistance and Elasticity

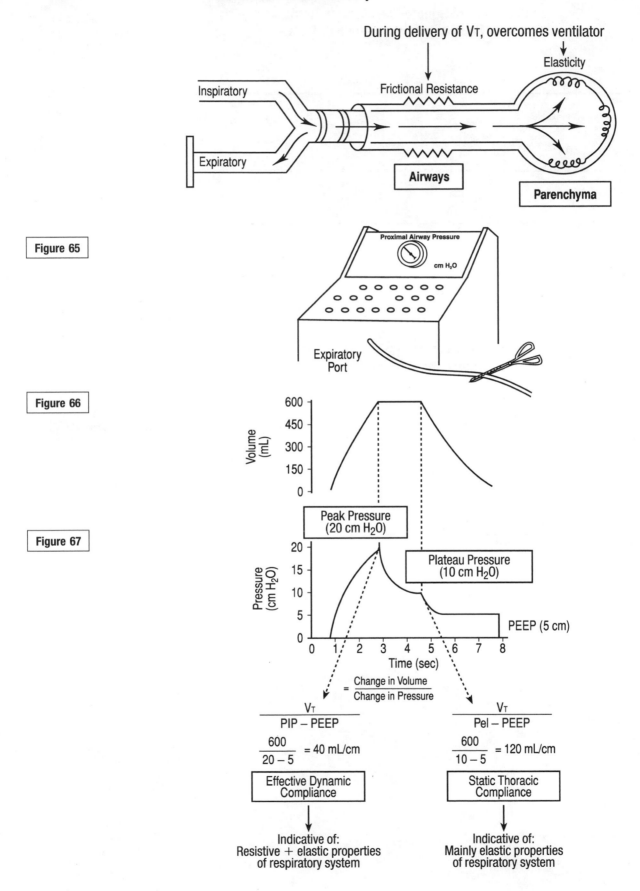

During delivery of VT, overcomes ventilator

Elasticity

Inspiratory

Frictional Resistance

Expiratory

Airways

Parenchyma

Proximal Airway Pressure

cm H₂O

Expiratory Port

$$= \frac{\text{Change in Volume}}{\text{Change in Pressure}}$$

Peak Pressure (20 cm H₂O)

Plateau Pressure (10 cm H₂O)

PEEP (5 cm)

$$\frac{V_T}{PIP - PEEP}$$

$$\frac{600}{20 - 5} = 40 \text{ mL/cm}$$

Effective Dynamic Compliance

Indicative of:
Resistive + elastic properties
of respiratory system

$$\frac{V_T}{Pel - PEEP}$$

$$\frac{600}{10 - 5} = 120 \text{ mL/cm}$$

Static Thoracic Compliance

Indicative of:
Mainly elastic properties
of respiratory system

Figure 64

Figure 65

Figure 66

Figure 67

Figure 68

Compliance—cont'd

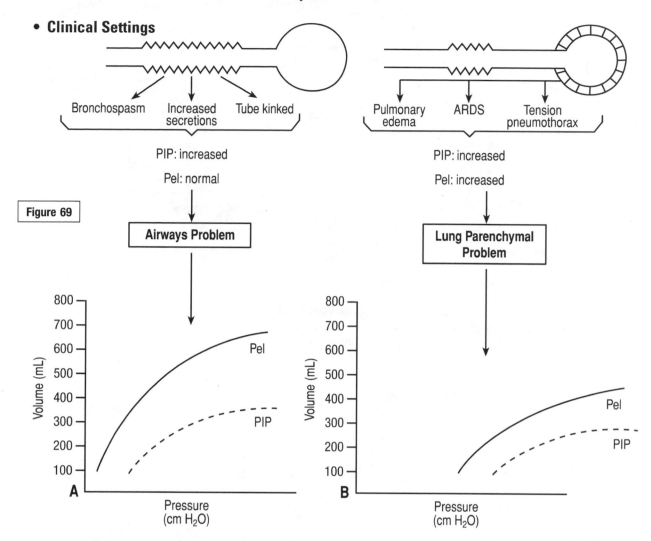

- **Clinical Settings**

Bronchospasm Increased secretions Tube kinked

Pulmonary edema ARDS Tension pneumothorax

PIP: increased

Pel: normal

Figure 69

Airways Problem

PIP: increased

Pel: increased

Lung Parenchymal Problem

A

Volume (mL) / Pressure (cm H$_2$O)

Pel

PIP

B

Volume (mL) / Pressure (cm H$_2$O)

Pel

PIP

- **Applications**
  1. Airways versus lung parenchymal problems
  2. Calculation of airways resistance
  3. Weaning index
  4. Predicting barotrauma
  5. Calculating optimal PEEP
  6. Calculating pressure support

Figure 70

Flow Rates and Inspiratory Time

- Effects

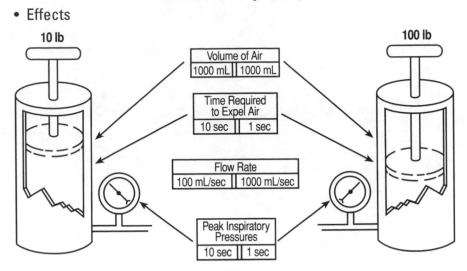

Figure 71

- **Example of Patient on Mechanical Ventilation**

(V_T = 1000 mL; peak flow rate = 1 L/sec [1000 mL/sec])
RR = 20/min—1 respiratory cycle = 3 sec

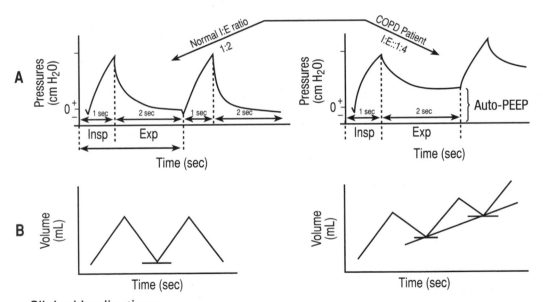

- Clinical Implications

	Low Peak Flows	High Peak Flows
Inspiration time	Prolonged	Shortened
Expiration time	Shortened	Lengthened
Peak pressures	Decreased	Increased
Patient's work of breathing	More	Less

Figure 72

Positive End-Expiratory Pressure

- **Alveoli (mid-end expiration)**

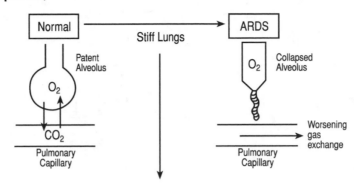

Figure 73

- **Treatment**

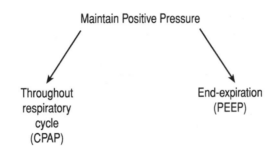

Figure 74

- **Configuration**

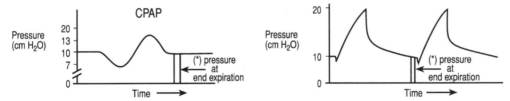

Figure 75

• **Effects of PEEP**

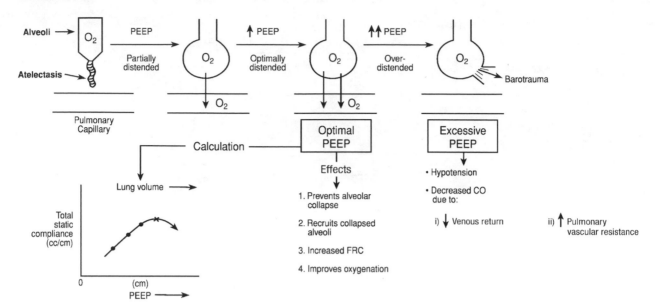

Calculation

Lung volume ⟶

Total
static
compliance
(cc/cm)

0   (cm)
        PEEP ⟶

**Optimal
PEEP**

Effects

1. Prevents alveolar
   collapse

2. Recruits collapsed
   alveoli

3. Increased FRC

4. Improves oxygenation

**Excessive
PEEP**

• Hypotension

• Decreased CO
  due to:

i) ↓ Venous return   ii) ↑ Pulmonary
                              vascular resistance

3. Commonly Used Formulae

Douglas Colquhoun, RRT
Linga Raju, MD

- *Resistance*. Driving pressure required to produce flow:

$$\text{Airway resistance} = \frac{\text{PIP} - \text{Pel (cm H}_2\text{O)}}{\text{Peak inspiratory flow rate (L/sec)}}$$

where

> PIP = peak inspiratory pressure
> Pel = plateau pressure
> Value: <10 cm H_2O/L/sec for mechanically ventilated patients

  - *Alveolar-arterial oxygen gradient*. Difference between alveolar and arterial partial pressure of oxygen:

$$P(A - a)O_2 = P_{AO_2} - P_{aO_2}$$

where

> P_{AO_2} = partial pressure of oxygen in alveolar gas
> P_{aO_2} = partial pressure of oxygen in arterial blood
> Value: <10 mm Hg on 21% oxygen
>   <50 mm Hg on 100% oxygen
>   Age correction = 2 + age/5
> Altered by: right-to-left shunt
> $\dot{V}/\dot{Q}$ mismatch
>   Diffusion impairment
>   Low mixed venous P_{O_2}

- *Alveolar gas equation*. Provides a close estimation of mean alveolar P_{O_2}, which will estimate what the P_{AO_2} should be:

$$P_{AO_2} = [(PB - PH_2O) \times F_{IO_2}] - P_{aCO_2}\left(F_{IO_2} + \frac{1 - F_{IO_2}}{RQ}\right)$$

where

> P_{AO_2} = partial pressure of oxygen in alveolar gas
> P_{aO_2} = partial pressure of oxygen in arterial blood
> P_{aCO_2} = partial pressure of carbon dioxide in arterial blood
> PB = barometric pressure (760 mm Hg)
> PH_2O = partial pressure of water (47 mm Hg)
> F_{IO_2} = fraction of inspired oxygen
> RQ = respiratory quotient
> Value: room air = 100 mm Hg
>   100% oxygen = 673 mm Hg

- *Alveolar ventilation*. The minute volume of gas that ventilates perfused alveoli:

$$\dot{V}_A = (V_T - V_D)f \qquad \text{and} \qquad P_{aCO_2} = K(\dot{V}_{CO_2}/\dot{V}_A)$$

where

> $\dot{V}_A$ = alveolar ventilation per minute
> V_T = tidal volume

147

$$\dot{V}_E = \text{minute ventilation}$$
$$\dot{V}_D = \text{dead space ventilation per minute}$$
$$f = \text{respiratory frequency}$$
$$\dot{V}_{CO_2} = CO_2 \text{ production/min}$$
$$\text{Value: 4–5 L/min}$$

Any changes in V_T, V_D, or frequency will alter $\dot{V}_A$.

Since

$$PaCO_2 = \frac{\dot{V}_{CO_2}}{(V_T - V_D) \times f} \times K$$

and

$$V_T \times f = \dot{V}_E$$

Then

$$PaCO_2 = \frac{\dot{V}_{CO_2}}{\dot{V}_E \left(1 - \dfrac{V_D \cdot f}{\dot{V}_E}\right)} \times K$$

$$= \frac{\dot{V}_{CO_2}}{\dot{V}_E \left(1 - \dfrac{V_D \cdot f}{V_T \cdot f}\right)} \times K$$

$$= \frac{\dot{V}_{CO_2}}{\dot{V}_E \left(1 - \dfrac{V_D}{V_T}\right)} \times K$$

- *Arterial/alveolar oxygen tension ratio.* Compares the arterial P_{O_2} with the alveolar P_{O_2} when the F_{IO_2} is altered. This ratio remains constant when F_{IO_2} is changed:

$$a/A\% = \frac{PaO_2}{PAO_2}$$

- *Arterial venous shunt equation.* Amount of blood that does not participate in gas exchange:

$$\dot{Q}s/\dot{Q}t = \frac{Cc'O_2 - CaO_2}{Cc'O_2 - C\overline{v}O_2}$$

where

$$\dot{Q}s/\dot{Q}t = \text{shunt fraction}$$
$$Cc'O_2 = \text{pulmonary end capillary oxygen content}$$
$$CaO_2 = \text{arterial oxygen content}$$
$$C\overline{v}O_2 = \text{mixed venous oxygen content}$$
Values: 2%–4% shunt is normal.
   Shunts >25% usually do not permit the PaO_2 to increase significantly when F_{IO_2} is increased.

- *Dynamic compliance.* Estimate of airways resistance and lung elasticity:

$$Cdyn = \frac{V_T \text{ (mL)}}{PIP - PEEP \text{ (cm } H_2O)}$$

where

   Cdyn = dynamic compliance
   PIP = peak inspiratory pressure
   PEEP = positive end-expiratory pressure
   Value: <50–70 mL/cm H_2O for patients on mechanical ventilation. This value is always lower than the static compliance value.

- *Static compliance.* Measurement of lung elasticity made at zero airflow (a true alveolar measurement):

$$Cdyn = \frac{V_T \ (mL)}{Pel - PEEP \ (cm \ H_2O)}$$

Value: 70–100 mL/cm H_2O on mechanical ventilation. Less than 25 mL/cm H_2O is an indication that the patient may not be ready to be weaned.

- *Fick equation.* Determining cardiac output by dividing oxygen consumption by the arteriovenous oxygen content difference:

$$\dot{Q}_T = \frac{\dot{V}_{O_2}}{(Ca_{O_2} - C\bar{v}_{O_2}) \times 10}$$

Value: 5 L/min

- *Inspiratory time.* Inspiratory time of a patient receiving mechanical ventilation:

$$T_I = \frac{V_T \ (mL)}{Flow \ rate \ (L/sec)}$$

- *Nitrogen balance*

N_2 balance = N_2 input − N_2 output − 2

$$N_2 \ input = \frac{amino \ acids \ or \ protein \ in \ grams/day}{6.25}$$

N_2 output = 24-hour excretion of urea nitrogen in urine plus addition of urea nitrogen to body water (as seen when BUN increases in serum)

−2 represents N_2 lost through skin, feces, sweat, and other excreta in which N_2 content is not routinely measured

Value: 0 ± 1 g/day (higher values represent anabolism [or lab error]; lower values are the hallmark of catabolism)

- *Oxygen consumption.* Amount of oxygen consumed per minute:

$$\dot{V}_{O_2} = \dot{Q}t \times C(a - \bar{v})_{O_2}$$

where

$\dot{Q}t$ = cardiac output
Ca_{O_2} = arterial oxygen content
$C\bar{v}_{O_2}$ = mixed venous oxygen content
Value: 225–275 mL/min

- *Oxygen content.* Amount of oxygen bound to hemoglobin plus amount of oxygen dissolved in plasma:

$$Ca_{O_2} = 1.34 \ mL \times Hb \ (g/dL) \times \frac{Sa_{O_2}}{100} + .003 \times Pa_{O_2}$$

$$C\bar{v}_{O_2} = 1.34 \ mL \times Hb \ (g/dL) \times \frac{S\bar{v}_{O_2}\% + 0.003}{100} \times P\bar{v}_{O_2}$$

Values: Ca_{O_2} (in arterial blood) = 20.7 mL O_2/dL blood
$\quad\quad\quad$ $C\bar{v}_{O_2}$ (in mixed venous blood) = 15.0 mL O_2/dL blood

Anemia, carbon monoxide poisoning, low hemoglobin, and methemoglobin all reduce oxygen content.

- *V_D/V_T ratio.* Ratio of the volume of air that does not participate in gas exchange to the tidal volume during quiet breathing:

$$V_D/V_T = \frac{Pa_{CO_2} - P\bar{E}_{CO_2}}{Pa_{CO_2}}$$

where

Pa_{CO_2} = partial pressure of arterial carbon dioxide
$P\bar{E}_{CO_2}$ = partial pressure of exhaled carbon dioxide
Value: normal = 0.33–0.45.

4. Case Studies

Faroque A. Khan, MB

Suhail Raoof, MD

CASE 1: STATUS ASTHMATICUS

A. A 20-year-old woman with asthma with a previous history of intubation and mechanical ventilation for asthma was admitted with severe shortness of breath. She was sweating profusely, was unable to complete sentences, and was tachypneic, using accessory muscles of respiration. Her vital signs were: BP of 140/90 mm Hg; pulse of 120 beats/min, RR of 30 breaths/min, and she had bilaterally decreased breath sounds. Her ABG revealed: pH of 7.20; $Paco_2$ of 46 mm Hg; Pao_2 of 89 mm Hg. Peak expiratory flow measured in the emergency room was 100 L/min. Chest radiograph was unremarkable.

What initial ventilatory management would be appropriate?

B. Despite appropriate medical therapy, the patient's PIP continued to rise to 60–70 cm. Her Pels were 30–40 cm and her ABG revealed a worsening anion gap metabolic acidosis as well as a respiratory acidosis (pH of 7.15; $Paco_2$ of 55 mm Hg, Pao_2 of 120 mm Hg). Additionally, progressive subcutaneous emphysema and a left pneumomediastinum were observed. A left chest tube was inserted. What management strategies can be used with this patient with complicated status asthmaticus who continues to have an elevated PIP?

C. Of the following parameters, which are predictive of successful weaning in a patient with severe status asthmaticus?
1. Oxygenation and ventilation.
2. Respiratory muscle strength.
3. Mechanics of ventilation.
    - VC, V_T
    - Dynamic compliance
    - RR

ANSWERS TO CASE 1

A. Type of ventilator: Volume-cycled positive-pressure usual—initially
   V_T: 500–600 mL (7–10 mL/kg)
   Mode: Assist/control
   RR: 10–12 breaths/min
   Fio_2:   0.4
   Flow rate: 60–80 L/min (monitor peak inspiratory pressures)
   Other: Sedate patient, and obtain and follow Cdyn and Cst
      information (i.e., peak and plateau pressures).

B. Change all ventilator settings to decrease PIP (decrease the V_T, decrease the flow rate, and sedate ± paralyze the patient). If hypoventilation ensues, use intravenous sodium bicarbonate to keep the pH at approximately 7.15. Continue to monitor the peak and plateau pressure difference. The following would be an example of the type of controlled hypoventilation that may be necessary for such a patient:

150

PIP (cm)	Pel (cm)	PIP-Pel (cm)	VT (mL)	Rate (breaths/min)	ABG pH/PaCO$_2$ (mmHg)/PaO$_2$ (mmHg)
					7.20/46/89
70	30	40	800	14	7.18/55/60*
55	25	30	600	10	7.25/60/65
40	25	15	600	10	7.39/42/62

* Give IV HCO$_3$.

C. Evaluate oxygenation and ventilation by the ABG. Oxygenation and ventilation must be normal at the time of weaning for status asthmaticus. CO$_2$ excretion must also be normal as evidenced by normal PaCO$_2$. Muscle strength is usually adequate with a peak negative effort significantly more than −25 cm. Ventilatory reserve is normal as well as the mechanics of respiration including the VC and VT. However, the dynamic compliance as generated from the peak pressure is initially high in status asthmaticus and must be markedly improved before extubation. The peak and plateau pressure difference should be approaching the normal range of approximately 10–15 cm. And finally, the ventilatory requirement should be such that the RR is significantly less than 30 cm, ideally less than 20 cm. Once the patient with status asthmaticus is ready for weaning and has fulfilled the above criteria, a rapid T-tube trial is usually successful.

CASE 2: CHRONIC OBSTRUCTIVE PULMONARY DISEASE

A. A 65-year-old heavy smoker with a 10-year history of COPD had a recent onset of an upper respiratory tract infection. He developed severe shortness of breath and worsening dyspnea while carrying groceries from the supermarket to his car. During his transport to the hospital, he was orally intubated with a size 8 ET-tube and was ventilated with a resuscitation bag by the transport team. His BP in the ambulance was 150/90 mm Hg and his pulse was 105 beats/min. In the emergency room, the patient was put on a volume ventilator with a VT of 800 mL, an RR of 15 breaths/min, a flow rate of 40 L/min, FIO$_2$ of 40%. His ABG revealed the following: pH of 7.32; PaCO$_2$ of 58 mm Hg; and PaO$_2$ of 60 mm Hg. Fifteen minutes later, his BP was 100/40 mm Hg with a pulse of 130 beats/min.

At this stage, which of the following would you consider?

1. Fluid resuscitation
2. Increasing FIO$_2$ and VT
3. Obtaining an emergent chest radiograph to look for pneumothorax
4. Administering thrombolytic therapy after demonstrating a massive pulmonary embolism
5. Occluding the expiratory port of the ventilator and checking for end-expiratory pressure.

B. By the second hospital day, the patient had stabilized with normal vital signs, and his ABG showed a pH of 7.36; a PaCO$_2$ of 55 mm Hg; and a PaO$_2$ of 80 mm Hg on 40% FIO$_2$. Weaning criteria, however, revealed the following: RR of 22 breaths/min; spontaneous VT of 250 mL (approximately 3 mL/kg); and maximum inspiratory pressure of −18 cm of H$_2$O. A T-piece weaning trial was attempted and the patient developed acute respiratory distress, sweating, and tachycardia, with an RR of 38 breaths/min. The ABG showed acute respiratory acidosis. Patient was put back on continuous mechanical ventilation in the assist/control mode and was re-evaluated for weaning.

What approach to maintenance mechanical ventilation and plans for weaning should be considered optimal in this patient with significant COPD and a tendency toward CO$_2$ retention?

A. In a patient with long-standing COPD, obstruction during the expiratory phase results in an I:E ratio of 1:3 to 1:5 or more. If such a patient is put on mechanical ventilation and given a large $\dot{V}E$ (at least 12 L in this case), he may develop auto-PEEP. Briefly, auto-PEEP or intrinsic PEEP develops when the time for exhalation is insufficient to allow the lungs to deflate to functional residual capacity (the resting lung volume) before the ventilator cycles the next breath.

Or, depicted mathematically, if this patient does not overbreathe the set rate, 15 breaths/min allows him 60/15 = 4 sec/breath. Now, with a flow rate of 40 L/min, 40/60 L of air can be delivered by the ventilator *per second,* i.e., 0.67 L/sec. So, to give a V_T of 800 mL (or 0.8 L), the ventilator will take 0.8/0.67 or approximately 1.2 sec. This will allow 2.8 sec for exhalation (4–1.2 sec). Thus I:E ratio will be 1.2:2.8 or 1:2.3 sec.

If the 1:E ratio is greater than 1:2.3, the patient will develop dynamic hyperinflation of the lungs as depicted below:

Figure 76

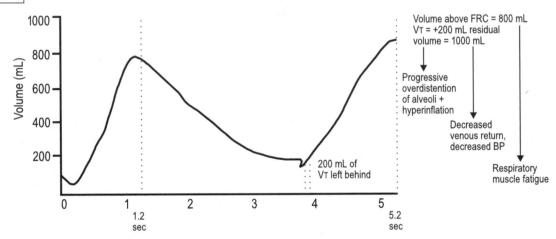

Of the options mentioned on p 151, the most appropriate would be (5) to occlude the expiratory port of the ventilator and check for end-expiratory pressure. If indeed it is determined that the patient has auto-PEEP, the following measures may be attempted:

1. Lowering the $\dot{V}E$ (decreased V_T, decreased RR if patient is not overbreathing the ventilator). Consider switching from assist/control mode to SIMV.
2. Increasing the flow rate from 40 L/min to 60 or 80 L/min. (This will cause the peak inspiratory pressures to increase.)
3. Bronchodilators—to decrease bronchospasm.
4. Sedation and paralysis, if necessary (for the agitated patient).
5. Adding PEEP (a few centimeters less than auto-PEEP).

B. Weaning criteria demonstrate a decreased spontaneous V_T (250 mL) and PImax (−18 cm). These parameters suggest respiratory muscle weakness. On the other hand, the patient was retaining CO_2 before the weaning trial. This implies that the dead space ventilation was increased. Hence the patient's $\dot{V}E$ requirements were high.

Figure 77

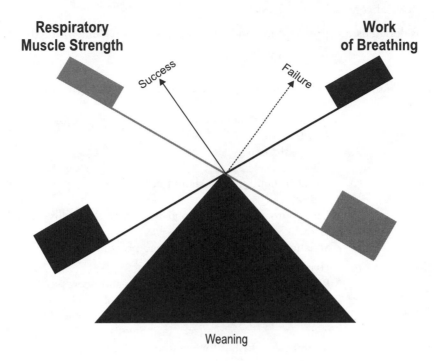

Respiratory Muscle Strength

Work of Breathing

Success

Failure

Weaning

Thus, the approach to be followed in the patient would be:
1. Allow more time for bronchospasm to resolve.
2. Allow the respiratory muscles to recover gradually.
3. Consider gradual weaning such as:
   • Pressure-support ventilation
   • Progressive IMV weaning

CASE 3: ADULT RESPIRATORY DISTRESS SYNDROME

A. A 34-year-old woman was admitted with chief complaints of fever, dry cough, shortness of breath, myalgias, and a vesicular skin eruption. She had been exposed to varicella 3 weeks earlier. On admission she was lethargic and covered with a typical varicella rash. She had a BP of 90/60 mm Hg; temperature of 102 °F; pulse of 130 beats/min; RR of 32 breaths/min; and her weight was 55 kg. The lungs revealed inspiratory rales. Chest radiograph showed extensive bilateral interstitial infiltrates, and her ABG on non-rebreather face mask revealed a pH of 7.48; $PaCO_2$ of 30 mm Hg; and PaO_2 of 54 mm Hg. She became progressively obtunded and was intubated.

What would be the appropriate ventilator settings and early management for this patient with ARDS?

B. The patient's oxygenation improved (PaO_2 of 68 mm Hg) on an FIO_2 of 70% and PEEP of 14 cm H_2O. During the next 72 hours, the patient developed a series of problems including:
1. Hypotension and tachycardia
2. A dilated endotracheal tube cuff
3. Radiographic appearance of a large subpleural air collection

What are the ventilator-associated causes of these problems as well as the strategies for resolving them?

C. By the tenth day in the hospital, the patient's infiltrates had remarkably improved and weaning from mechanical ventilation was planned.

What considerations must be kept in mind when weaning this patient with ARDS?

ANSWERS TO CASE 3

A. Type of ventilator: Volume-cycled, positive-pressure ventilator (pressure-targeted ventilator may also be used)

     V_T: 10 mL/kg initially; lower to 5–7 mg/kg, if possible

     Mode: Assist/control

     RR: 12 breaths/min

     FIO_2:   1.0

     Flow rate: 40–60 L/min initially (should not be less than patient's intrinsic inspiratory flow)

     PEEP: One approach would be to give 5 cm H_2O initially; then 1–2 cm above lower inflection point

     Other: Sedation, follow peak and plateau pressures.

B. 1. Problem: Hypotension/tachycardia.

     Cause: PEEP can lead to decreased preload and decreased CO with resultant hypotension and tachycardia. PEEP of greater than 15 cm H_2O may additionally decrease LV compliance and may decrease coronary blood flow.

     Solution: *Noninvasive*: Listen for breath sounds. Monitor compliance. Determine lower inflection point.

         Invasive: Hemodynamic monitoring with a pulmonary artery catheter to evaluate optimal PEEP by following CO, PAOP, and $S\bar{v}O_2$.

         Therapy (applies to invasive only): Increase intravascular volume and, later, begin administering vasopressor drugs, if indicated. Inverse ratio ventilation with pressure control has been used in ARDS patients in whom conventional ventilator therapy fails.

     2. Problem: Enlarged ET-tube cuff—i.e., cuff/trachea ratio (a cuff trachea ratio of >1.5:1)

     Cause: Inadvertent overinflation of the ET-tube cuff leads to increased cuff pressures, decreased tracheal capillary perfusion, and tracheal ischemia. Tracheomalacia, tracheoesophageal fistula, and tracheal stenosis can occur.

     Solution: Observe the cuff/trachea ratio daily on the chest radiograph. Maintain cuff pressure <20 cm of H_2O. Use minimal air leak technique. Reintubate with a longer ET-tube, especially if there is a large cuff/trachea ratio as well as large air leak leading to hypoventilation.

     3. Problem: Pneumothorax.

     Cause: Mechanical ventilation and PEEP-induced volutrauma. Pulmonary interstitial gas can collect in localized pockets under the visceral pleura leading to a large collection of gas visible on the chest radiograph.

     Solution: Decrease PEEP if possible; decrease V_T, if possible. Sedate and paralyze patient. Prepare for urgent chest tube insertion.

C. ARDS is a form of hypoxic respiratory failure. Evaluation of expected oxygenation is therefore necessary after extubation.
- FIO_2 should be <50%.
- PEEP must be minimal (≤5 cm H_2O).
- PaO_2 must be >60 mm Hg.
- PaO_2/FIO_2 >200, if possible.
- Oxygen delivery should be at a maximum (e.g., optimize CO, Hb).

A possible method of weaning when all of the above are fulfilled is a fairly rapid weaning trial with T-piece or IMV.

CASE 4: CHRONIC OBSTRUCTIVE PULMONARY DISEASE

A. A 72-year-old man with COPD has the following baseline parameters:

ABG (room air): pH of 7.37; $PaCO_2$ of 60 mm Hg; PaO_2 of 62 mm Hg. The patient's HCO_3 on the fluid balance was 35 mEq/L.

He is admitted with exacerbation of his underlying respiratory disorder.

His ABG on admission reveals a pH of 7.16; $PaCO_2$ of 86 mm Hg; PaO_2 of 36 mm Hg. The patient is intubated and mechanically ventilated with the assist/control mode at a rate of 20 breaths/min; V_T of 800 mL; and FIO_2 of 0.6.

Thirty minutes later, he appears confused and starts seizing.

What is the reason for the seizures?
What ventilatory management would be appropriate?

B. His condition stabilizes. Four days later, he is ready to be weaned.

His ABG on assist/control at a rate of 10 breaths/min; V_T of 700 mL; FIO_2 of 40% reveals the following:

pH of 7.38; $PaCO_2$ of 46 mm Hg; PaO_2 of 84 mm Hg; and HCO_3 of 28.

What are the problems expected in weaning this patient? What are the solutions?

ANSWERS TO CASE 4

A. The seizures are caused by posthypercapnic metabolic alkalosis.

The ABG reveals a pH of 7.58; $PaCO_2$ of 35 mm Hg; and a PaO_2 of 85 mm Hg.

Give enough $\dot{V}E$ to keep the $PaCO_2$ and pH at the patient's baseline. (In this case, the $PaCO_2$ was approximately 60 mm Hg and the pH was 7.37). To determine the appropriate $\dot{V}E$ in this case (i.e., to achieve a baseline $PaCO_2$ of 60 mm Hg):

$$\dot{V}E(1) \times PaCO_2(1) = \dot{V}E(2) \times PaCO_2(2)$$
$$(20 \times .8) \times 35 = \dot{V}E(2) \times 60$$
$$\dot{V}E(2) = 16 \times 35/60 \text{ Approximately } 9.0 \text{ L}$$

Since

$$RR \times V_T = \dot{V}E$$
$$V_T = 9000 \text{ mL}/800 \text{ mL} = 10 \text{ breaths/min}$$

B. On extubation, the patient will retain $PaCO_2$ to approximately 60 mm Hg.

To retain HCO_3, renal compensation will take approximately 2–3 days (from 28 to 35).

Problems to be expected:

1. Increased $PaCO_2$: Alveolar hypoventilation, atelectasis, increased $\dot{V}/\dot{Q}$ mismatch, further hypoxemia.

2. Uncompensated respiratory acidosis: pH will decrease to approximately 7.26.

   Allow the $PaCO_2$ to increase gradually over a 2- to 3-day period to baseline by progressively decreasing $\dot{V}E$ before extubating patient.

CASE 5: LEFT VENTRICULAR FAILURE

A 65-year-old man with COPD and LVF is admitted with acute respiratory failure. He has been mechanically ventilated for 1 week. His clinical condition has improved. Spontaneous ventilatory parameters currently are: V_T of 350 mL; VC of 900 mL; RR of 30 breaths/min; and PI max $= -45$ cm H_2O. The $\dot{V}E$ while on the ventilator is 10.5 L/min. ABG (RA) reveals pH of 7.36; $PaCO_2$ of 46 mm Hg; PaO_2 of 68 mm Hg. The HR is 98 beats/min, and the PAOP is 10 mm Hg. A T-piece trial is given.

The trial is terminated at 30 minutes owing to tachycardia, tachypnea, diaphoresis, and an increase in a $PaCO_2$ to 60 mm Hg.

What is the most likely explanation for the failure to wean?

Patients with COPD and LVF have been described as developing acute respiratory failure when extubated. As a result of sudden removal of mechanical ventilation, the following causal mechanisms have been implicated:

1. Decreased intrathoracic volume → decreased intrathoracic pressure → increased venous return → increased preload → pulmonary edema
2. Ischemia → decreased contractility of myocardium
3. Increased systemic BP + decreased pleural pressure → increased afterload

In a study of 15 patients with COPD, Lemaire and colleagues (1988) showed that the following changes took place upon extubation:

	Pre-extubation	Post-extubation
1. Esophageal pressure (cm H_2O)	+5	−2
2. Cardiac index	3.2	4.3
3. Mean systemic BP (mm Hg)	77	90
4. HR (beats/min)	97	112
5. PAOP (cm H_2O)	8	25
6. Pa_{CO_2} (mm Hg)	42	58

Thus, these patients should be diuresed and kept on mechanical ventilation until their volume status has been corrected. Positive-pressure ventilation serves to decrease venous return, which is beneficial in patients with LVF. Sudden removal from the ventilator facilitates venous return and may worsen LVF, resulting in failure to wean.

5. Compliance Measurement Exercise

Faroque A. Khan, MB
Suhail Raoof, MD

A. **A patient with acute respiratory failure is intubated and put on a mechanical ventilator. The ventilator settings are as follows:**

Assist/control mode	
V_T	600 mL
F_{IO_2}	100%
PEEP	5 cm H_2O
The following pressures were recorded:	
PIP	65 cm H_2O
Pel	55 cm H_2O

Calculate the following: 1) Cdyn characteristics
2) Cst characteristics

B. Match the following:

	Compliance	
	Dynamic (mL/cm H_2O)	Static (mL/cm H_2O)
(a)	75	80
(b)	20	60
(c)	20	25

1. Normal respiratory system
2. Bronchial intubation
3. Pulmonary emboli
4. Bronchospasm
5. ARDS

Answers to Compliance Questions

A. 1) Dynamic compliance $= \dfrac{V_T}{PIP - PEEP} = \dfrac{600}{65 - 5} = 10$ mL/cm

2) Static compliance $= \dfrac{V_T}{Pel - PEEP} = \dfrac{600}{55 - 5} = 12$ mL/cm

B.   1. a
2. c
3. a
4. b
5. c

6. Quiz

A. Basic concepts
Robert M. Kacmarek, PhD

1. During pressure-control ventilation, when end-expiratory flow is zero prior to the end of the inspiratory phase:
   a. The tidal volume can be increased by increasing inspiratory time.
   b. The peak airway pressure equals the end-inspiratory plateau pressure.
   c. The pressure control level should be increased.
   d. The inspiratory time is excessive.

2. The primary advantage of pressure-control ventilation over volume-control ventilation is:
   a. The peak alveolar pressure is constant.
   b. The tidal volume is constant.
   c. Oxygenation is improved.
   d. Hemodynamics are improved.

3. During pressure-control ventilation, increasing inspiratory time increases the tidal volume if:
   a. No auto-PEEP is present.
   b. The peak alveolar pressure is <35 cm H_2O.
   c. The delivered flow at end inspiration is greater than zero.
   d. The rate is <20/min.

4. Which one of the following statements about the differences between auto-PEEP and applied PEEP in the management of oxygenation during adult respiratory distress syndrome is true?
   a. Local lung unit total PEEP levels differ.
   b. The functional residual capacity of lung units with short time constants increases more with applied PEEP than with auto-PEEP.
   c. Overdistention of lung units with long time constants is greater with auto-PEEP than with applied PEEP.
   d. Hemodynamic compromise is greater with the same level of auto-PEEP than with applied PEEP.

5. Which one of the following is *not* considered a primary pathophysiologic indication for mechanical ventilation?
   a. Apnea
   b. Acute respiratory failure
   c. Impending acute respiratory failure
   d. Increased work of breathing

B. Types of ventilators
Robert M. Kacmarek, PhD

6. Which one of the following is *not* a primary difference between positive-pressure and negative-pressure ventilation?
   a. Method of application
   b. Ability to assist ventilation
   c. Overall efficacy of ventilatory support
   d. Delivery of supplemental oxygen

7. The primary reason leaks occur with full-face mask noninvasive positive-pressure ventilation is:
   a. Mask brand
   b. Mask size
   c. Airway pressure that is too high
   d. Use of PEEP

8. Which one of the following is *not* a potential contraindication to noninvasive positive-pressure ventilation?
   a. Respiratory arrest
   b. Inability to protect the airway
   c. Inability to clear secretions
   d. $Paco_2 \geq 80$ mm Hg
9. Pressure support on ICU ventilators should *not* be used with nasal masks because of:
   a. Gastric distention
   b. Flow cycling to exhalation
   c. Lack of a back-up rate
   d. Inadequate inspiratory time
10. Which one of the following is *not* an advantage of ICU ventilators over portable pressure ventilators during acute administration of noninvasive positive-pressure ventilation?
    a. Precise Fio_2 control
    b. Monitoring of patients' rate, volume, and system pressure
    c. Variety of modes
    d. More effective ventilation

C. Initial ventilatory support
Suhail Raoof, MD
Douglas Colquhoun, RRT
11. Which of the following sets of ventilator settings would be appropriate initial settings for a 70-kg patient with severe hypoxemic respiratory failure?

Ventilation	Oxygen	Tidal volume
Assist/control, 14	100%	700 mL
Assist/control, 25	40%	1.0 L
Assist/control, 8	40%	500 mL
Synchronized intermittent mandatory ventilation	35%	700 mL

12. During volume ventilation, the most common cause of a lag in the increase of the peak airway pressure is:
    a. Peak inspiratory flow rate that is too high
    b. Peak inspiratory flow rate that is too low
    c. Development of auto-PEEP
    d. Shortened inspiratory phase
13. Which of the following sets of conditions is the likely result of higher inspiratory flow rates?
    a. Higher peak inspiratory pressures, longer inspiratory time, reduced work of breathing by patient, higher incidence of auto-PEEP
    b. Lower peak inspiratory pressures, shorter inspiratory time, increased work of breathing by patient, lower incidence of auto-PEEP
    c. Higher peak inspiratory pressures, shorter inspiratory time, decreased work of breathing by patient, lower incidence of auto-PEEP

D. Modes of ventilation + PEEP
Suhail Raoof, MD
Douglas Colquhoun, RRT
14. Which of the following statements about pressure support is *not* correct?
    a. It is used to overcome airway resistance.
    b. It augments patients' spontaneous tidal volume.
    c. It is indicated in patients without spontaneous inspiratory effort.
15. Indications for PEEP therapy include:
    a. Decreased Pao_2 with increased Fio_2
    b. Decreased compliance
    c. Presence of auto-PEEP
    d. All of the above

16. Ventilator changes that would reduce or eliminate auto-PEEP include
    a. Decrease of the set tidal volume
    b. Decreased tidal volume frequency
    c. Increased tidal volume peak flow rate
    d. Addition of low levels of PEEP
    e. All of the above

E. Compliance studies
Suhail Raoof, MD
Douglas Colquhoun, RRT

17. In a patient on mechanical ventilation, bronchodilator therapy would likely cause which of the following effects?
    a. Deceased peak airway pressure
    b. Increased peak airway pressure
    c. Decreased plateau pressure
    d. Increased plateau pressure
18. In a patient who develops pneumothorax on mechanical ventilation, which of the following changes are expected to occur?
    a. Increase in peak inspiratory pressures
    b. Decrease in plateau pressure
    c. Increase in dynamic compliance
    d. Increase in static compliance
19. A 60-kg man at a tidal volume of 500 mL, PIP of 65 cm H_2O, plateau pressure of 35 cm H_2O, and an inspiratory flow rate of 60 L/min has an auto-PEEP of 15 cm H_2O. Which of the following is *not* true of this patient?
    a. Dynamic compliance of 10 mL/cm, static compliance of 40 mL/cm
    b. Dynamic compliance that is high and static compliance that is normal
    c. Airways resistance of 30 cm/L/sec
    d. Airways resistance and a respiratory system compliance problem

F. Weaning questions
Raymond Lavery, RRT

20. The most common cause of increase in CO_2 when nutritional supplementation is begun during weaning is:
    a. Muscle fatigue
    b. Excessive administration of carbohydrate calories
    c. Decreasing the SIMV rate too quickly
    d. Excessive pressure support
21. Which one of the following does *not* facilitate weaning a patient from mechanical ventilation?
    a. Adding appropriate nutritional support early during mechanical ventilation
    b. Monitoring ventilatory reserve parameters frequently
    c. Using a small diameter endotracheal tube to increase work of breathing performed by the respiratory muscles
    d. Getting the patient out of bed to chair as early as possible
22. Which of the following statements about weaning from mechanical ventilation is *not* true?
    a. A negative inspiratory force of >20–25 cm H_2O is usually a good indication of respiratory muscle strength.
    b. A vital capacity of <15 mL/kg is adequate for successful weaning.
    c. Volume overload contributes to difficulty in weaning patients from mechanical ventilation.
    d. Patients requiring long-term ventilation may benefit from synchronized intermittent mandatory ventilation with pressure support when weaning is initiated.

G. Neuromuscular diseases, cardiac disorders

Raymond Lavery, RRT

Linga Raju, MD

23. Which one of the following conditions does *not* typically occur in patients with ventilatory failure due to neuromuscular disease?
    a. Normal ventilatory drive
    b. Normal inspiratory muscle strength
    c. Near normal lung function
    d. Predisposition to develop atelectasis from inadequate lung inflation

24. In patients with neuromuscular disease, which one of the following statements about ventilatory management is true?
    a. Negative-pressure ventilation is more effective than positive-pressure ventilation.
    b. Low tidal volume (5 to 7 mL/kg) should be used.
    c. The risk of barotrauma is higher than in patients with intrinsic lung disease.
    d. Affected patients are more comfortable with high inspiratory flow rates (>60 L/min).

25. Which one of the following statements about the cardiovascular effects of mechanical ventilation (PPV) is *not* true?
    a. Increased intrathoracic pressure always results in decreased cardiac output.
    b. Mechanical ventilation may decrease venous return by decreasing pressure gradient from peripheral veins to the right atrium.
    c. Mechanical ventilation may increase right ventricular afterload by increasing the resistance of the pulmonary vessels.
    d. Mechanical ventilation may decrease left ventricular filling.
    e. Mechanical ventilation may increase stroke volume and hence cardiac output by reducing wall stress and afterload of a dilated failing left ventricle that is operating on the flat/depressed portion of the cardiac function curve.

26. In patients with myocardial ischemia, which one of the following statements is *not* true?
    a. Increased work of breathing and hence the increased oxygen demand may adversely affect the myocardial oxygen supply/demand relationship.
    b. Myocardial ischemia may decrease compliance of the left ventricle and cause diastolic dysfunction.
    c. Increasing pulmonary capillary pressure and decreasing lung compliance may result in increased work of breathing and create a vicious circle.
    d. Spontaneous ventilation with an increase in the spontaneous work of breathing is likely to be beneficial.

27. In postoperative patients, which one of the following statements is *not* true?
    a. Anesthetic-induced decrease in functional residual capacity coupled with thoracic or upper abdominal incision predisposes to atelectasis.
    b. Variable period of mechanical ventilation is required depending upon the residual effects of anesthetic agents, narcotics, and muscle relaxants.
    c. Concern is to avoid iatrogenic complications of unnecessary prolonged mechanical ventilation.
    d. Prospective studies have proven that mechanical ventilation is beneficial in stabilizing a more physiologic cardiopulmonary status in the postoperative period.

H. Terminal weaning

Ashok Karnik, MD

28. A 52-year-old woman is hospitalized with an exacerbation of her severe COPD. Therapy with antibiotics, bronchodilators, and supplemental oxygen is begun. Measurement of arterial blood gases shows a pH of 7.30, $PaCO_2$ of 69 mm Hg, and PaO_2 of 44 mm Hg. Intubation and mechanical ventilation are indicated. The patient's family urges intubation, but the patient, who is alert, oriented, and seems to understand the consequences of her decision, refuses intubation.
    What is an appropriate action at this time?
    a. Intubate and ventilate the patient.
    b. Sedate the patient and then intubate her.
    c. Ask the hospital attorney to get a court order and then intubate the patient.
    d. Continue current management and comfort measures.
    e. Get permission from the court to withhold assisted ventilation.

29. Which one of the following statements about the persistent vegetative state is true?
    a. The PVS results from damage to the brain stem nuclei.
    b. Patients in a PVS are awake but unaware of their surroundings.
    c. Patients in a PVS have spontaneous eye movement and can follow a moving object.
    d. Patients in a PVS have no recognizable language.
    e. Patients in a PVS have no legal rights because they have lost their "personhood."
30. A 60-year-old man sustained anoxic brain damage during cardiac arrest. He remains on mechanical ventilation for 2 months without improvement in his clinical condition. Under which of the following conditions may terminal weaning be done in this patient?
    a. You believe that it is futile to continue the management in this patient.
    b. The hospital administration fears that this patient is occupying a bed that can be better used for a younger, more acutely ill patient.
    c. The patient's insurance company refuses to pay his bills.
    d. A health care proxy appointed by the patient requests you to do so.
    e. The wife of the patient who has been giving consents during the patient's illness requests you to withdraw the ventilator. No other health care proxy is available and the patient's wishes regarding this matter are not known.

I. Mechanical ventilation therapy of ARDS
Raymond Lavery, RRT
31. PEEP is indicated in patient with ARDS to:
    a. Improve oxygenation with a lower FIO_2
    b. Decrease cardiac output
    c. Overdistend functional alveoli
    d. Increase the work of breathing in the spontaneously breathing patient.
32. Pressure-control ventilation is usually considered in ARDS when:
    a. Peak airway pressures are below 30 cm H_2O
    b. Peak airway pressures are greater than 40 cm H_2O
    c. The patient is ready to be weaned
    d. Patients require an FIO_2 of >0.50
33. When inverse ratio ventilation is used in patients with ARDS:
    a. Sedation and paralysis are usually necessary
    b. Pressure-control ventilation cannot be used
    c. A short inspiratory time is recommended
    d. It is not necessary to monitor auto-PEEP
34. Patients with ARDS may benefit from permissive hypercapnia because:
    a. Hypoxia may be corrected
    b. Acute lung injury may be prevented
    c. Auto-PEEP may be increased
    d. Barotrauma may be minimized

J. COPD
Liziamma George, MD
35. Which one of the following statements about auto-PEEP in mechanically ventilated patients is *most* correct?
    a. Increasing the rate and minute ventilation is likely to offer significant benefit.
    b. End-expiratory pressure may be higher in the alveoli than measured at mouth.
    c. Auto-PEEP can be ruled out by observing the pressure reading on the manometer of the ventilator at end expiration.
    d. The most frequent clinical manifestation of auto-PEEP is depression of diaphragm.
36. Which one of the following is *most likely not* a clinical sign of severe asthma?
    a. Absence of wheezing
    b. Subcutaneous emphysema
    c. Pulsus paradoxus >15 mm Hg
    d. Dyspnea that precludes speech
    e. Metabolic alkalosis

37. A 25-year-old man presents with severe status asthmaticus. Despite therapy with high doses of β_2-agonists and corticosteroids, he requires mechanical ventilation for respiratory muscle fatigue. Appropriate ventilator settings include:
   a. High respiratory rates (20-25 breaths/min)
   b. Low inspiratory flow rates
   c. PEEP (10 cm H_2O)
   d. Small tidal volumes

38. A 30-year-old man is intubated for status asthmaticus. Arterial blood gas measurement on FIO_2 of 0.4, VT of 600 mL, RR of 18 breaths/min, and inspiratory flow rate of 60 L/min. ABG revealed a pH of 7.16, $PaCO_2$ of 70 mm Hg, and PaO_2 of 95 mm Hg. Peak airway pressure is 80 cm H_2O. The auto-PEEP is 15 cm H_2O. Further adjustment in VT or rate failed to improve $PaCO_2$ or auto-PEEP. Which one of the following measures would *not* be appropriate in this patient?
   a. Sedation and muscle relaxation
   b. Add PEEP, 10 cm H_2O
   c. Consider bicarbonate infusion
   d. Reduction of inspiratory flow rate

Quiz Answers

1.	B	20.	B
2.	A	21.	C
3.	C	22.	B
4.	D	23.	B
5.	D	24.	D
6.	C	25.	A
7.	B	26.	D
8.	D	27.	D
9.	B	28.	D
10.	D	29.	B,D
11.	A	30.	D
12.	B	31.	A
13.	C	32.	B
14.	C	33.	A
15.	D	34.	D
16.	E	35.	B
17.	A	36.	E
18.	A,C	37.	D
19.	A,B	38.	A

GLOSSARY

ABG	Arterial blood gas
A/C	Assist/control mechanical ventilation
ADL	Aid to daily living
ADP	Adenosine diphosphate
ALS	Amyotrophic lateral sclerosis
APACHE	Acute Physiologic and Chronic Health Evaluation Scoring System
APRV	Airway pressure release ventilation
ARDS	Acute respiratory distress syndrome
ATP	Adenosine triphosphate
BiPAP	Bilevel pressure ventilation
BP	Blood pressure
CaO_2	Arterial oxygen content
CcO_2	Pulmonary end capillary oxygen content
Cdyn	Dynamic compliance of respiratory system
CHF	Congestive heart failure
CHO	Carbohydrate
Cst	Static compliance of respiratory system
CMV	Controlled mode ventilation
CNS	Central nervous system
COPD	Chronic obstructive pulmonary disease
CPAP	Continuous positive airway pressure
CROP	Compliance, rate, oxygenation, pressure (integrative weaning index)
CVA	Cerebrovascular accident
$C\bar{v}O_2$	O_2 content of mixed venous blood
CVS	Cardiovascular system
$D(A-a)O_2$	Alveolar arterial oxygen gradient
$\dot{D}O_2$	Oxygen delivery or oxygen transport/min
DP	Driving pressure
ECMO	Extracorporeal membrane oxygenation
$ECCO_2R$	Extracorporal CO_2 removal
EMG	Electromyography
EPAP	End-expiratory positive airway pressure
ET-tube	Endotracheal tube
f	Frequency of respiration
FEV_1	Forced expiratory volume in one second
FIO_2	Fractional concentration of oxygen in inspired gas
$f$mv	Ventilator rate
FRC	Functional residual capacity
HCO_3	Bicarbonate
HFJV	High-frequency jet ventilation
HFO	High-frequency oscillation
HFPPV	High-frequency positive-pressure ventilation
HFV	High-frequency ventilation
HR	Heart rate
ICP	Intracranial pressure
IMV	Intermittent mandatory ventilation
IPAP	Inspiratory positive airway pressure
IPPB	Intermittent positive pressure breathing
IRV	Inverse ratio ventilation
IVOX	Intravascular blood gas exchange (or intravascular oxygen exchange system)
LFPPV	Low-frequency positive-pressure ventilation
LV	Left ventricular
LVF	Left ventricular failure
mm Hg	Millimeters of mercury
MMV	Mandatory minute ventilation

MVV	Maximum voluntary ventilation
NIPPV	Noninvasive positive-pressure ventilation
NPV	Negative-pressure ventilation
P 0.1	Airway occlusion pressure measured at 0.1 seconds of occlusion
$PaCO_2$	Partial pressure of carbon dioxide in arterial blood
$PaCO_2$ mv	$PaCO_2$ on the ventilator
PaO_2	Partial pressure of oxygen in arterial blood
PAO_2	Partial pressure of oxygen in alveolar gas
Palv	Alveolar pressures
PAOP	Pulmonary artery occlusion pressure (or, pulmonary capillary pressure)
$\overline{PAP}$	Mean pulmonary artery pressure
PAV	Proportional assist ventilation
$P\overline{aw}$	Mean airway pressure
P_B	Barometric pressure
PCO_2	Partial pressure of carbon dioxide
PC-IRV	Pressure-control inverse ratio ventilation
PCV	Pressure-control ventilation
PCWP	Pulmonary capillary wedge pressure (or, pulmonary artery occlusion pressure)
$PECO_2$	Partial pressure of exhaled carbon dioxide
PEEP	Positive end-expiratory pressure
PEF	Peak expiratory flow rate
Pel	Plateau pressure
Pemax	Maximum expiratory pressure
$P\overline{E}CO_2$	Partial pressure of exhaled carbon dioxide
PH_2O	Partial pressure of water
PImax	Maximum inspiratory pressure
PIO_2	Partial pressure of oxygen in the inspired gas
PIF	Peak inspiratory flow
PIP	Peak inspiratory pressure
PO_2	Partial pressure of oxygen
Ppl	Pleural pressure
PPV	Positive-pressure ventilation
prn	pro re nata [L] as the occasion arises, as necessary
PSV	Pressure-support ventilation
P–V curve	Pressure–volume curve
$P\overline{v}O_2$	Partial pressure of oxygen in the mixed venous blood
$\dot{Q}s/\dot{Q}t$	Shunt fraction
Raw	Airway resistance
REE	Resting energy expenditure
RQ	Respiratory quotient
RR	Respiratory rate
RV	Right ventricular
SaO_2	Oxygen saturation in arterial blood
SIADH	Syndrome of inappropriate antidiuretic hormone
SIMV	Synchronized intermittent mandatory ventilation
$S\overline{v}O_2$	Saturation of hemoglobin in the mixed venous blood
SvO_2	Mixed venous oxygen saturation
T_E	Expiratory time
T_I	Inspiratory time
Ti/Tot	Ratio of inspiratory time to the total respiratory cycle (duty cycle)
TLC	Total lung capacity
TPN	Total parenteral nutrition
V_A	Alveolar ventilation
$\dot{V}_A$	Alveolar ventilation per minute
VAP	Ventilator-associated pneumonia
VC	Vital capacity
VCV	Volume-controlled ventilation

VCV-IRV	Volume-controlled inverse ratio ventilation
V_{CO_2}	Volume of carbon dioxide (STPD) production per minute
V_D	Volume dead air space
$\dot{V}_D$	Dead space ventilation per minute
V_D/V_T	Ratio of dead space volume to tidal volume
$\dot{V}_E$	Minute ventilation
$\dot{V}_{O_2}$	Oxygen consumption per unit of time
$\dot{V}/\dot{Q}$	Ventilation-perfusion ratio
V_T	Tidal volume
WI	Weaning index
WOB	Work of breathing

Annotated Bibliography

General Aspects of Mechanical Ventilation

Consensus Conference on the Essentials of Mechanical Ventilation. Respir Care. 1992;37:999–1130.

Morganroth ML, ed. Mechanical ventilation. Clin Chest Med. 1988;9:1–173.

Nahum A, Marini J. Recent advances in mechanical ventilation. Clin Chest Med. 1996;17(3).

Perel A, Stock MC. Handbook of mechanical ventilatory support. Williams and Wilkins; 1992:3–80.

Pierson DJ. Indications for mechanical ventilation in acute respiratory failure. Respir Care. 1983;28:570–8.

"Special Issue" Conference on Mechanical Ventilation, Parts I and 2, Respir Care, Vol. 32, No. 6 and 7, 1987.

Slutsky AS. American College of Chest Physicians Conference on Mechanical Ventilation. Chest. 1993;104:1833–59.

Tobin MJ, ed. Mechanical ventilation. Crit Care Clin. 1990;489–805.

Eight comprehensive and up-to-date reviews covering all aspects of mechanical ventilation, including conventional and new modes of mechanical ventilation, indications, complications, and approaches to weaning.

Modes of Ventilation

Synchronized Intermittent Mandatory Ventilation

Giuliani R, Mascia L, Reccia F, et al. Patient-ventilator interaction during synchronized intermittent mandatory ventilation: effects of flow triggering. Am J Respir Crit Care Med. 1995;151:1–9.
Study demonstrating that flow triggering reduces inspiratory effort during mandatory and spontaneous SIMV and obtains a better patient–ventilator interaction.

Groeger JS, Levinson MR, Carlon GC. Assist control versus synchronized intermittent mandatory ventilation during acute respiratory failure. Crit Care Med. 1989;17:607–12.
No evidence was found to support any clear-cut advantage of SIMV versus assist/control in the management of respiratory failure.

Hudson LD, Hurlow RS, Craig CK, et al. Does intermittent mandatory ventilation correct respiratory alkalosis in patients receiving assisted mechanical ventilation? Am Rev Respir Dis. 1985;132:1071–4.
This study suggests that the patients' underlying condition and respiratory efforts, not the selection of mode, contributed to the development of respiratory alkalosis.

Sassoon CS, Del Rosario N, Fei R, et al. Influence of pressure- and flow-triggered synchronous intermittent mandatory ventilation on inspiratory muscle work. Crit Care Med. 1994;22:1933–41.
Study showing that during SIMV, the method of ventilator triggering has a significant effect on the total work rate and inspiratory muscle work of spontaneous breathing.

Weisman IM, Rinaldo JE, Rogers RM, et al. Intermittent mandatory ventilation. Am Rev Respir Dis. 1983;127:641–7.
An excellent review of the historical perspective of IMV, as well as an evaluation of the punitive advantages and disadvantages of IMV.

Amato MB, Barbas CS, Bonassa J, et al. Volume-assured pressure support ventilation (VAPSV). A new approach for reducing muscle workload during acute respiratory failure. Chest. 1992;102:1225–34.

This study reports the preliminary clinical evaluation of a new mode of ventilation → volume assured pressure support ventilation (VAPSV), which incorporates PSV with conventional volume assisted cycles.

Ambrosino N, Nava S, Bertone P, et al. Physiologic evaluation of pressure support ventilation by nasal mask in patients with stable COPD. Chest. 1992;101:385–91.

Banner MJ, Kirby RR, Kirton OC, et al. Breathing frequency and pattern are poor predictors of work of breathing in patients receiving pressure support ventilation. Chest. 1995;108:1338–44.

Demonstrates that work of breathing should be measured directly because variables of breathing pattern commonly used at bedside appear to be inaccurate and misleading inferences of the work of breathing.

Black JW, Grover BS. A hazard of pressure support ventilation. Chest. 1988;93:333–5.

Brochard L, Harf A, Lorina H, et al. Inspiratory pressure support prevents diaphragmatic fatigue during weaning from mechanical ventilation. Am Rev Respir Dis. 1989;139:513–21.

Optimal levels of pressure support ventilation were shown to prevent the development of diaphragmatic fatigue.

Brochard L, Pluskiwa F, Lemaire F. Improved efficacy of spontaneous breathing with inspiratory pressure support. Am Rev Respir Dis. 1987;136:411–5.

A pressure support of 10 cm H_2O improved VT, oxygenation, and $PaCO_2$ and decreased respiratory rate and transdiaphragmatic pressures as compared with a continuous flow system and spontaneous breathing through the demand valve. This study demonstrated reduced work during spontaneous breathing using PSV.

Cohen IL, Bilen Z, Krishnamurthy S. The effects of ventilator working pressure during pressure support ventilation. Chest. 1993;103:588–92.

Describes the consequence of altering ventilator pressures on airway pressure and flow characteristics during PSV.

Harding J, Kemper M, Weissman C. Pressure support ventilation attenuates the cardiopulmonary response to an acute increase in oxygen demand. Chest. 1995;107:1665–72.

A study showing the role of PSV in attenuating the pulmonary and hemodynamic responses to interventions that increase oxygen ordered.

Hughes CW, Popovich J. Uses and abuses of pressure support ventilation. J Crit Illness. 1989;4:25–32.

Jounieaux V, Duran A, Levi-Valensi P. Synchronized intermittent mandatory ventilation with and without pressure support ventilation in weaning patients with COPD from mechanical ventilation [published erratum appears in Chest. 1994;106:984]. Chest. 1994;105:1204–10.

A prospective study comparing two weaning modalities in COPD patients requiring mechanical ventilation. SIMV appeared very useful in weaning COPD patients from MV. PSV marginally reduced the weaning period.

Kreit JW, Capper MW, Eschenbacher WL. Patient work of breathing during pressure support and volume-cycled mechanical ventilation. Am J Respir Crit Care Med. 1994;149:1085–91.

A study showing that patient work of breathing during PSV may be greater than, less than, or equal to the work performed during volume-cycled mechanical ventilation.

Lofaso F, Brochard L, Touchard D, et al. Evaluation of carbon dioxide rebreathing during pressure support ventilation with airway management system (BiPAP) devices. Chest. 1995;108:772–8.

A study showing evidence that significant CO_2 rebreathing occurs with standard BiPAP systems and this drawback can be overcome by using a non-rebreathing valve.

MacIntyre NR. Respiratory function during pressure support ventilation. Chest. 1986;89:677–83.

A discussion and presentation of evidence that PSV can influence patient comfort, ventilatory pattern, and work of breathing.

MacIntyre NR. Pressure support ventilation: effects on ventilatory reflexes and ventilatory muscle workloads. Respir Care. 1987;32:447–56.

MacIntyre NR. Weaning from mechanical ventilatory support: volume assisting intermittent breaths versus pressure assisting every breath. Respir Care. 1988;33:121–5.

Useful comparison of the quantity and quality of patient work as well as patient synchrony on the ventilator during weaning with IMV as compared to PSV.

Marini JJ, Capps JS, Culver BH. The inspiratory work of breathing during assisted mechanical ventilation. Chest. 1985;87:612–8.

Study demonstrating that inspiratory muscles continue to expend energy throughout inspiration even when subjects were put on the assist/control mode of mechanical ventilation.

Meecham Jones DJ, Paul EA, Jones PW, et al. Nasal pressure support ventilation plus oxygen compared with oxygen therapy alone in hypercapnic COPD. Am J Respir Crit Care Med. 1995;152:538–44.

A comparison of nasal PSV and oxygen with oxygen alone in patients with COPD showing that there is significant improvement in daytime arterial PaO_2 and $PaCO_2$, total sleep time, sleep efficiency, and overnight $PaCO_2$ after nasal pressure support ventilation plus oxygen as compared with oxygen alone.

Shelledy DC, Rau JL, Thomas-Goodfellow L. A comparison of the effects of assist-control, SIMV, and SIMV with pressure support on ventilation, oxygen consumption, and ventilatory equivalent. Heart Lung. 1995;24:67–75.

A study to quantify the ventilator efficiency of different modes of mechanical ventilation such as SIMV with PSV, SIMV, and assist/control.

Tokioka H, Saito S, Saeki S, et al. The effect of pressure support ventilation on auto-PEEP in a patient with asthma. Chest. 1992;101:285–6.

Inverse Ratio Ventilation

Lessard MR, Guerot E, Lorino H, et al. Effects of pressure-controlled with different I:E ratios versus volume-controlled ventilation on respiratory mechanics, gas exchange, and hemodynamics in patients with adult respiratory distress syndrome. Anesthesiology. 1994;80:983–91.

A prospective controlled study, showing no short-term beneficial effects of PCV or PC-IRV over conventional VCV with PEEP in patients with ARDS.

Manthous CA, Schmidt GA. Inverse ratio ventilation in ARDS. Improved oxygenation without auto-PEEP. Chest. 1993;103:953–4.

A case report showing improved oxygenation on IRV in a patient with ARDS without auto-PEEP.

Shanholtz C, Brower R. Should inverse ratio ventilation be used in adult respiratory distress syndrome? Am J Respir Crit Care Med. 1994;149:1354–8.

Sydow M, Burchardi H, Ephraim E, et al. Long-term effects of two different ventilatory modes on oxygenation in acute lung injury. Comparison of airway pressure release ventilation and volume-controlled inverse ratio ventilation. Am J Respir Crit Care Med. 1994;149:1550–6.

Valta P, Takala J. Volume-controlled inverse ratio ventilation: effect on dynamic hyperinflation and auto-PEEP. Acta Anesthesiol Scand. 1993;37:323–8.

The effects of IRV and PEEP on dynamic hyperinflation and auto-PEEP are studied in sedated, paralyzed patients with ARDS and in postoperative patients after coronary artery bypass grafting.

High-frequency Ventilation

Fort P, Farmer C, Westerman J, et al. High-frequency oscillatory ventilation for adult respiratory distress syndrome: a pilot study. Crit Care Med. 1997;25:937–47.

A safety and efficacy study using high-frequency oscillation in ARDS.

Positive End-Expiratory Pressure

Gattinoni L, Pesenti A, Avalli L, et al. Pressure volume curve of total respiratory system in acute respiratory failure: computed tomographic scan study. Am Rev Respir Dis. 1987;136:730–6.

Shapiro BA, Cane RD, Harrison RA. Positive end-expiratory pressure therapy in adults with special reference to acute lung injury: a review of the literature and suggested clinical correlations. Crit Care Med. 1984;12:127–41.

Excellent summary of mechanisms and complications of PEEP.

Weisman IM, Rinaldo JE, Rogers RM. Current concepts positive end expiratory pressure in adult respiratory failure. N Engl J Med. 1982;307:1381–4.

Concise and well-written summary of the uses for PEEP and a rational approach to PEEP application.

Noninvasive Positive-Pressure Ventilation in Acute Respiratory Failure

Bach JR, Alba A. Management of chronic alveolar hypoventilation by nasal ventilation. Chest. 1990;97:52–7.

Back JR, Alba A, Bohatiuk G, et al. Mouth intermittent positive pressure ventilation in the management of postpolio respiratory insufficiency. Chest. 1987;91:859–64.

DiMarco AF, Connors AF, Altose MD, et al. Management of chronic alveolar hypoventilation with nasal positive pressure breathing. Chest. 1987;92:950–4.

Ellis ER, Bye PT, Druderer JW, et al. Treatment of respiratory failure during sleep in patients with neuromuscular disease: positive-pressure ventilation through a nose mask. Am Rev Respir Dis. 1987;135:148–52.

Ellis ER, Grumstein RR, Chan S, et al. Noninvasive ventilatory support during sleep improves respiratory failure in kyphoscoliosis. Chest. 1988;94:811–5.

Gay PC, Patel AM, Viggiano RW, et al. Nocturnal nasal ventilation for treatment of patients with hypercapnic respiratory failure. Mayo Clin Proc. 1991;66:695–703.

Hill NS, Eveloff SE, Carlisle CC, et al. Efficacy of nocturnal nasal ventilation in patients with restrictive thoracic disease. Am Rev Respir Dis. 1992;145:365–71.

Strumpf DA, Carlisle CC, Millman RP, et al. An evaluation of the Respironics BiPAP Bi-Level CPAP Device for Delivery of Assisted Ventilation. Respir Care. 1990;35(5): 415–22.

Waldhoen RE. Nocturnal nasal intermittent positive pressure ventilation with bi-level positive airway pressure (BiPAP) in respiratory failure. Chest. 1992;101:516–21.

Chronic Obstructive Pulmonary Disease

Celli B, Lee H, Criner G, et al. Controlled trial of external negative pressure ventilation in patients with severe airflow limitation. Am Rev Respir Dis. 1989;140:1251–6.

Cropp A, Dimarco AF. Effects of intermittent negative pressure ventilation on respiratory muscle function in patients with severe chronic obstructive pulmonary disease. Am Rev Respir Dis. 1987;135:1056–61.

Scano G, Gigliotti F, Duranti R, et al. Changes in ventilatory muscle function with negative pressure ventilation in patients with severe COPD. Chest. 1990;97:322–7.

Acute Respiratory Failure

Brochard L, Isabey D, Piquet J, et al. Reversal of acute exacerbation of chronic obstructive lung disease by inspiratory assistance with a face mask. N Engl J Med. 1990;323:1523–30.

A study evaluating the efficacy of a noninvasive ventilatory assistance apparatus to provide inspiratory pressure support by means of a face mask.

Brochard L, Mancebo J, Wysocki M, et al. Noninvasive ventilation for acute exacerbations of chronic obstructive pulmonary disease. N Engl J Med. 1995;333:871–22.

Chevrolet JC, Jolliet P, Abajo B, et al. Nasal positive pressure ventilation in patients with acute respiratory failure. Chest. 1991;100:775–82.

Hill NS. Noninvasive ventilation: does it work, for whom, and how? Am Rev Respir Dis. 1993;147:1050–5.

An excellent review article on NIPPV describing the effectiveness of NIV in chronic and acute respiratory failure.

Jasmer RM, Luce JM, Matthay MA. Noninvasive positive pressure ventilation for acute respiratory failure. Underutilized or overrated? Chest. 1997;111:1672–8.

Meduri GU. Noninvasive positive pressure ventilation in patients with acute respiratory failure. Clin Chest Med. 1996;17:513–53.

Meduri GU, Abou-Shala N, Fox RC, et al. Noninvasive face mask mechanical ventilation in patients with acute hypercapnic respiratory failure. Chest. 1991;100:445–54.

A study indicating that mechanical ventilation via face mask is a viable option for short-term ventilatory support of patients with hypercapnic respiratory failure.

Meduri GU, Turner RE, et al. Noninvasive positive pressure ventilation via face mask: first-line intervention in patients with acute hypercapnic and hypoxemic respiratory failure. Chest. 1993;109:179–93.

A report on the effectiveness of NIPPV in correcting gas exchange abnormalities and avoiding intubation.

Rosenberg JI, Goldstein RS. Noninvasive positive pressure ventilation: a positive view in need of supportive evidence. Chest. 1997;111:1479–82.

Wysocki M, Tric L, Wolff MA, et al. Noninvasive pressure support ventilation in patients with acute respiratory failure: a randomized comparison with conventional therapy. Chest. 1995;107:761–8.

Newer Techniques of Ventilation and Oxygenation

Abraham E, Yoshihara G. Cardiorespiratory effects of PC-IRV in severe respiratory failure. Chest. 1989;96:1356–9.

Patients with severe ARDS were switched to PC-IRV owing to failure to oxygenate with conventional ventilation. As expected, there was a decrease in PIP and improvement in oxygenation. There was no change in mean arterial pressure, cardiac index, oxygen delivery and consumption, and other hemodynamic parameters.

Cameron PD, Oh TE. Newer modes of mechanical ventilatory support. Anaesth Intensive Care 1986;14:258–66.

Cane RD, Peruzzi WT, Shapiro BA. Airway pressure release ventilation in severe acute respiratory failure. Chest. 1991;100:460–3.

Carlon GC, Miodownik S, Ray CJ, et al. Technical aspects and clinical implications of high frequency jet ventilation with a solenoid valve. Crit Care Med. 1981;947–50.

Carlon GC, Howland WS, Ray C, et al. High frequency jet ventilation: a prospective randomized evaluation. Chest. 1983;84:551–9.

Chang HK. Mechanisms of gas transport during ventilation by high frequency oscillation. J Appl Physiol. 1984;56:553–63.

Couser JL Jr, Make BJ. Transtracheal oxygen decreases inspired minute ventilation. Am Rev Respir Dis. 1989;139:627–31.

Downs JB, Stock MC. Airway pressure release ventilation: a new concept in ventilatory support. Crit Care Med. 1987;15:459–61.

Summarizes the basic principles of APRV and theoretical advantages.

Froese AB, Bryan AC. High frequency ventilation: state of the art. Am Rev Respir Dis. 1987;135:1363–74.

Garner W, Downs JB, Stock MC, et al. Airway pressure release ventilation (APRV): a human trial. Chest. 1988;94:779–81.

A study using APRV in 14 patients who underwent bypass surgery. APRV was found to support ventilation in patients with oxygenation, V_E, and hemodynamic measures similar to those achieved when controlled ventilation was used.

Gurevitch MJ, Van Dyke J, Young ES, et al. Improved oxygenation and lower peak airway pressure in severe adult respiratory distress syndrome: treatment with inverse ratio inhalation. Chest. 1986;89:211–3.

A study of two patients showing the possible uses of IRV in ARDS.

Hewlett AM, Platt AS, Terry VG. Mandatory minute volume. Anesthesia. 1977;32:163–9.

Kacmarek RM, Hess D. Pressure controlled inverse ratio ventilation: panacea or auto-PEEP? Respir Care. 1990;35:945–8.

Lain DC, DiBenedetto R, Morris SL, et al. Pressure control inverse ratio ventilation as a method to reduce peak inspiratory pressure and provide adequate ventilation and oxygenation. Chest. 1989;95:1081–8.

A total of 19 patients with ARDS or pneumonia with high PIP, F_{IO_2}, or PEEP on conventional ventilation were switched to PC-IRV. This resulted in an increase in PaO$_2$ and MAP, with decreases in PIP, F_{IO_2}, or PEEP on conventional ventilation.

Mackey DF, Shykoff BE, et al. Transtracheal insufflation of O$_2$ has no effect on minute ventilation in chronic respiratory failure (abstract). Chest. 1990;98:114S.

Marantz S, Patrick W, Webster K, et al. Respiratory response to different levels of proportional assist (PAV) in ventilator-dependent patients. Am Rev Respir Dis. 1992; 145:A525.

Marcy TW, Marini JJ. Inverse ratio ventilation in ARDS. Chest. 1991;100:494–504.

Review of current status of IRV. This article discusses risks of volume-controlled and pressure-controlled ventilators. It elucidates some of the risks, including barotrauma, drop in cardiac output, need for sedation and paralysis (owing to patient discomfort), conceptual difficulties in changing frequency to change alveolar ventilation, and lack of controlled studies.

Poelaert JI, Vogelaers D, Colardyn FA. Evaluation of the hemodynamic and respiratory effects of inverse ratio ventilation with a right ventricular ejection fraction catheter. Chest. 1991;99:1444–50.

Patients with ARDS (n = 15) were started on IRV at an I:E ratio of 1:1, which was gradually increased to 4:1. A right ventricular ejection fraction PA catheter identified two subgroups of patients. The first group of "respondees" demonstrated preload dependence and developed an increase in cardiac index on IRV. The group of non-respondees were afterload dependent and had a drop in oxygen delivery while on IRV.

Rasanen J. IMPRV: synchronized APRV, or more? Intensive Care Med. 1992;18:65–6.

Rasanen J, Downs JB, Stock MC. Cardiovascular effects of conventional positive pressure ventilation and airway pressure release ventilation. Chest. 1988;93:911–5.

Slutsky AS. American College of Chest Physicians Consensus Conference on Mechanical Ventilation. Chest. 1993;104:1833–59.

Smith DW, Frankel LR, Ariagno RL. Disassociation of mean airway pressure and lung volume during high-frequency ventilation. Crit Care Med. 1988;16:531–5.

Spofford B, Christopher K, et al. Transtracheal oxygen therapy: a guide for the respiratory therapist. Respir Care. 1987;32:345–52.

Stock MC, Downs JB. Airway pressure release ventilation: a new approach to ventilatory support during acute lung injury. Respir Care. 1987;32:517–24.

APRV is a pressure-limited mode of ventilation that resembles IRV but differs by allowing spontaneous breathing. Patients are maintained at a present level of "CPAP" for the entire respiratory cycle except for a specific period (1.5 second) when the airway pressure is released.

Stock MC, Downs JB, Frolicher DA. Airway pressure release ventilation. Crit Care Med. 1987;15:462–6.

Tharratt RS, Allen RP, Albertson TE. Pressure controlled inverse-ratio ventilation in severe adult respiratory failure. Chest. 1988;94:755–62.

An uncontrolled trial of PC-IRV that shows safety and the possible benefit of this mode of therapy in ARDS.

Wissing DR, Romero MD, George RB. Comparing the newer modes of mechanical ventilation: a guide to design advances and specific clinical applications. J Crit Illness. 1987;2:41–9.

A very practical review of new modes in mechanical ventilation including pressure support, high-frequency IRV, and others.

Younes M. Proportional assist ventilation: a new approach to ventilatory support. Theory. Am Rev Respir Dis. 1992;145:114–20.

Younes M, Puddy A, Roberts D, et al. Proportional assist ventilation: results of an initial clinical trial. Am Rev Respir Dis. 1992;145:121–9.

A new approach to mechanical ventilation in which the ventilatory assistance is determined by spontaneous inspiratory flow rate and V_T. This approach appears to be more physiologic than most other modes of mechanical ventilation currently available.

Monitoring During Mechanical Ventilation

Bone RC. Diagnosis for causes of acute respiratory distress by pressure volume curves. Chest. 1976;70:740–6.

Bone RC. Monitoring ventilatory mechanics in acute respiratory failure. Respir Care. 1983;28:597–603.

The original and follow-up article stating the method and clinical use of the pressure volume curves in respiratory failure.

Dreyfuss D, Soler P, Basset G, et al. High-inflation pressure pulmonary edema: respective effects of high airway pressure, high tidal volume, positive end-expiratory pressure. Am Rev Respir Dis. 1988;137:1159–64.

Glauser FL, Polatty RC, Sessler CN. Worsening oxygenation in the mechanically ventilated patient: causes, mechanisms, and early detection. Am Rev Respir Dis. 1988;138:458–65.

Kollef MH, Shapiro SD, Silver P, et al. Initial experience with a central respiratory monitoring unit as a cost-saving alternative to the intensive care unit for Medicare patients who require long-term ventilator support. Chest. 1988;93:395–7.

Lemaire F, Teboul JL, Cinotti L, et al. Acute left ventricular dysfunction during unsuccessful weaning from mechanical ventilation. Anesthesiology. 1988;69:171–9.

Milic-Emili J. How to monitor intrinsic PEEP—and why. J Crit Illness. 1992;7:25–32.

Pepe PE, Marini JJ. Occult positive end-expiratory pressure in mechanically ventilated patients with airflow obstruction: the auto-PEEP effect. Am Rev Respir Dis. 1982; 126:166–70.

Initial report of auto-PEEP (intrinsic PEEP), explaining mechanisms, diagnosis, and management.

Rossi A, Gottfried SB, Zocchi L, et al. Measurement of static compliance of the total respiratory system in patients with acute respiratory failure during mechanical ventilation: the effect of intrinsic positive end-expiratory pressure. Am Rev Respir Dis. 1985;131: 672–7.

A discussion of the adverse effects of auto-PEEP on hemodynamics and weaning in patients with respiratory failure.

Scott LR, Benson MS, Pierson DJ. Effect of inspiratory flow rate and circuit compressible volume on auto-PEEP during mechanical ventilation. Respir Care. 1986;31:1075–8.

A two-part study comparing a laboratory model and a clinical evaluation of various flow rates and the effect on auto-PEEP. Authors conclude that the highest inspiratory flow rates and a low compressible volume circuit are effective in reducing auto-PEEP.

Tobin MJ. Respiratory monitoring in the intensive care unit. Am Rev Respir Dis. 1988; 138:1625–42.

Intrinsic Positive End-Expiratory Pressure

Appendini L, Patessio A, Zanaboni S, et al. Physiologic effects of positive end-expiratory pressure and mask pressure support during exacerbation of chronic obstructive pulmonary disease. Am J Respir Crit Care Med. 1994;149:1069–76.

Brandolese R, Broseghini C, Pokse G, et al. Effects of intrinsic PEEP on pulmonary gas exchange in mechanically-ventilated patients. Eur Resp J. 1993;6:358–63.

Fleury B, Murciano D, Talamo C, et al. Work of breathing in patients with chronic obstructive pulmonary disease in acute respiratory failure. Am Rev Respir Dis. 1985;131:822–7.

Gay PC, Rodarte JR, Hubmayer RD. The effects of positive expiratory pressures on isovolume flow and dynamic hyperinflation in patients receiving mechanical ventilation. Am Rev Respir Dis. 1989;139:621–6.

Gottfried SB, Reissman H, Ranieri VM. A simple method for the measurement of intrinsic positive end-expiratory pressure during controlled and assisted modes of mechanical ventilation. Crit Care Med. 1992;20(5):621–9.

Milic-Emili J. How to monitor intrinsic PEEP—and why. J Crit Illness. 1992;7:25–32. *These articles describe intrinsic PEEP, and elaborate its effects on pulmonary gas exchange measurement of intrinsic PEEP in mechanically ventilated patients.*

Ranieri VM, Grasso S, Fiore T, et al. Auto-positive end-expiratory pressure and dynamic hyperinflation. Clin Chest Med. 1996;(17):379–94.

Rossi A, Polese G, Brandi G, et al. Intrinsic positive end-expiratory pressure (PEEPi) [Review]. Intensive Care Med. 1995;21:522–36.

ARDS and PEEP

Dirusso SM, Nelson LD, Safcsak K, Miller RS. Survival in patients with severe adult respiratory distress syndrome treated with high-level positive end-expiratory pressure. Crit Care Med. 1995;23:1485–96.

Eissa NT, Ranieri VM, Corbeil C, et al. Effect of PEEP on the mechanics of the respiratory system in ARDS patients. J Appl Physiol. 1992;73:1728–35.

Seven excellent articles that describe the mechanisms, physiologic alterations, chest wall mechanics, and complications of PEEP in patients with ARDS.

Gattinoni L, Pelosi P, Crotti S, et al. Effects of positive end-expiratory pressure on regional distribution of tidal volume and recruitment in adult respiratory distress syndrome. Am J Respir Crit Care Med. 1995;151:1807–14.

Pelosi P, Cereda M, Foti G, et al. Alterations of lung and chest wall mechanics in patients with acute lung injury: effects of positive end-expiratory pressure. Am J Respir Crit Care Med. 1995;152:531–7.

Ranieri VM, Mascia L, Fiore T, et al. Cardiorespiratory effects of positive end-expiratory pressure during progressive tidal volume reduction (permissive hypercapnia) in patients with acute respiratory distress syndrome. Anesthesiology. 1995;83:710–20.

Schuster DP, Howard DK. The effect of positive end-expiratory pressure on regional pulmonary perfusion during acute lung injury. J Crit Care. 1994;9:100–10.

Valta P, Takala J, Eissa NT, et al. Does alveolar recruitment occur with positive end-expiratory pressure in adult respiratory distress syndrome patients? J Crit Care. 1993;8(1):34–42.

COPD and PEEP

Appendini L, Patessio A, Zanaboni S, et al. Physiologic effects of positive end-expiratory pressure and mask pressure support during exacerbations of chronic obstructive pulmonary disease. Am J Respir Crit Care Med. 1994;149:1069–76.

Georgopoulos D, Giannouli E, Patakas D. Effects of extrinsic positive end-expiratory pressure on mechanically ventilated patients with chronic obstructive pulmonary disease and dynamic hyperinflation. Intensive Care Med. 1993;19:197–203.

Two articles dealing with the physiological effects of PEEP in patients with COPD.

Weaning from Mechanical Ventilation

Arnold JH, Truog RD, Thompson JE, et al. High-frequency oscillatory ventilation in pediatric respiratory failure. Crit Care Med. 1993;21:272–8.

Brochard L, Rauss A, Benito S, et al. A comparison of three methods of gradual withdrawal from ventilatory support during weaning from mechanical ventilation. Am J Respir Crit Care Med. 1994;150:896–903.

Duration of weaning with PSV was 5.7 ± 3.7 days as compared to IMV (9.9 ± 8.2 days) and with trials of spontaneous breathing (8.5 ± 8.3 days).

Esteban A, Frutos F, Tobin MJ, et al. A comparison of four methods of weaning patients from mechanical ventilation. N Engl J Med. 1995;332:345–50.

Once-daily trial of spontaneous breathing led to extubation about three times more quickly than SIMV and twice as quickly as PSV.

Esteban A, Alía I, Gordo F, et al. Extubation outcomes after spontaneous breathing trials with T-tube or pressure support ventilation. Am J Respir Crit Care Med. 1997;156:459–65.

Hall JB, Wood LDH. Liberation of patient from mechanical ventilation. JAMA. 1987;257:1621–8.

Jabour ER, Rabil DM, Truwrit JD, et al. Evaluation of a new weaning index based on ventilatory endurance and the efficacy of gas exchange. Am Rev Respir Dis. 1991;144:531–7.

Kirton OC, DeHaven CB, Morgan JP, et al. Elevated imposed work of breathing masquerading as ventilator weaning intolerance. Chest. 1995;108:1021–5.

Kollef MH, Shapiro SD, Silver P, et al. A randomized, controlled trial of protocol-directed versus physician-directed weaning from mechanical ventilation. Crit Care Med. 1997;25:567–74.

Levy MM, Miyasaki A, Langston D. Work of breathing as a weaning parameter in mechanically ventilated patients. Chest. 1995;108:1018–20.

Linton DM, Potgieter PD, Davis S, et al. Automatic weaning from mechanical ventilation using an adaptive lung ventilation controller. Chest. 1994;106:1843–50.

Scoggin CH. The technique of weaning from mechanical ventilation. J Crit Illness. 1986;1:59–69.

Practical tips on weaning from mechanical ventilation, including trouble shooting when weaning is not routine.

Tobin MJ, Perez W, Guenther SM, et al. Pattern of breathing during successful and unsuccessful trials of weaning from mechanical ventilation. Am Rev Respir Dis. 1986; 134:1111–8.

An excellent prospective comparison of patients who were successfully weaned with those who were not. Specifically, multiple physiologic parameters were evaluated and the development of hypercapnia was found to be associated with simultaneous development of rapid, shallow breathing.

Tomlinson JR, Miller KS, Lorch DG, et al. A prospective comparison of IMV and T-piece weaning from mechanical ventilation. Chest. 1989;96:348–52.

Terminal Withdrawal of Mechanical Ventilation from Patients in Persistent Vegetative States

American Thoracic Society. Position Paper. Withholding and withdrawing life-sustaining therapy. Ann Intern Med. 1991;115:478–85.

Bone RC, Rackow EC, Weg JG, and members of the ACCP/SCCM Consensus Panel. Ethical and moral guidelines for the initiation, continuation and withdrawal of intensive care. Chest. 1990;97:949–58.

Campbell ML, Carlson RW. Terminal weaning from mechanical ventilation: ethical and practical considerations for patient management. Am J Crit Care. 1992;3:52–6.

Council of Scientific Affairs and Council on Ethical and Judicial Affairs. Persistent vegetative state and the decision to withdraw or withhold life support. JAMA. 1990;263:426–30.

Daly BJ, Newlon B, Montenegro HD, Langdon T. Withdrawal of mechanical ventilation: ethical principles and guidelines for terminal weaning. Am J Crit Care. 1993;2: 217–23.

Nelson WA, Bernat JL. Decisions to withhold or terminate treatment. Neurol Clin. 1989;7:759–74.

NIH Workshop Summary. Withholding and withdrawing mechanical ventilation. Am Rev Respir Dis. 1986;134:1327–30.

American College of Physicians Ethics Manual. Ann Intern Med. 1992;117:947–60.

Ruark JE, Raffin TA. Initiating and withdrawing life support: principles and practice in adult medicine. N Engl J Med. 1988;318:25–30.

Schneiderman LJ, Spragg RG. Ethical decisions in discontinuing mechanical ventilation. N Engl J Med. 1988;318:984–8.

Weir RF, Gostin L. Decisions to abate life sustaining treatment for nonautonomous patients. JAMA. 1990;264:1846–53.

Complications of Mechanical Ventilation

Bennett J, Brachman P, ed. Hospital infections. Boston: Little, Brown; 1992.

Panlilio AL, Culves DH, Gaynes RP, et al. Methicillin-resistant *Staphylococcus aureus* in US hospital, 1975–1991. Infect Control Hosp Epidemiol. 1992;13:582–6.

Centers for Disease Control. Guidelines for preventing transmission of Mycobacterium tuberculosis in health-care facilities. Fed Regist. 1994;59:54242–303.

Centers for Disease Control. Recommendations for preventing the spread of vancomycin resistance. MMWR Morb Mortal Wkly Rep. 1995;44:1–13.

Centers for Disease Control. Guidelines for prevention of intravascular device-related infections (Notice). Federal Register. 1995;60:49978–50006.

Craven DE, Kunches LM, Kilinsky V, et al. Risk factors for pneumonia and fatality in patients receiving continuous mechanical ventilation. Am Rev Respir Dis. 1986;133:792–6.
A review of the risk factors for pneumonia in ventilated patients including the problem of gastric prophylaxis and nosocomial pneumonia.

Fagon JY, Chastre J, Domart Y, et al. Nosocomial pneumonia in patients receiving continuous mechanical ventilation. Am Rev Respir Dis. 1989;139:877–84.

Gammon BR, Shin MS, Buchalter SE, et al. Pulmonary barotrauma in mechanical ventilation. Patterns and risk factors. Chest. 1992;102:2;568–72.

Pinsky MR. The effects of mechanical ventilation on the cardiovascular system. Crit Care Clin. 1990;6:663–78.

Sahn SA, Lakshminarayan S, Petty TL. Weaning from mechanical ventilation. JAMA. 1976;235:2208–12.

Tablan OC, Anderson LJ, Arden NH, et al. Guidelines for prevention of nosocomial pneumonia. The Hospital Infection Control Practices Advisory Committee, Centers for Disease Control and Prevention. Infect Control Hosp Epidemiol. 1994;9:588–627.

Tsuna K, Miura K, Takeya M, et al. Histopathologic pulmonary changes from mechanical ventilation at high peak airway pressures. Am Rev Respir Dis. 1991;143:1115–20.
Study showing that pulmonary parenchymal injury results from mechanical ventilation in experimental animals with peak inspiratory pressures of 40 cm H_2O. No injury was seen in control animals ventilated with PIP of 18 cm H_2O.

Valles J, Artigas A, Rello J, et al. Continuous aspiration of subglottic secretions in preventing ventilator-associated pneumonia. Ann Intern Med. 1995;122:179–86.

Wollschlager CM, Conrad AR, Khan FA. Common complications in critically ill patients. Dis Mon. 1988;34:221–93.
A comprehensive review of complications in ICU patients including the complications of respiratory failure and mechanical ventilation.

Zwillich CW, Pierson DJ, Creagh CE, et al. Complications of assisted ventilation: a prospective study of 354 consecutive episodes. Am J Med. 1974;57:161–70.
The classic prospective study of ventilator complications.

Nutrition in the Mechanically Ventilated Patient

Askanazi J, Weissman C, Rosenbaum SH, et al. Nutrition and the respiratory system. Crit Care Med. 1982;10:163–72.

Cerra FB, Cheung NK, Fischer JE, et al. Disease-specific amino acid infusion (FO[80]) in hepatic encephalopathy: a prospective randomized double-blind controlled trial. JPEN J Parenter Enteral Nutr. 1985;9:288–95.
Seventy-five patients with hepatic encephalopathy were prospectively randomized. Use of branched-chain amino acid–enriched solution was very effective even if high protein was used.

Grant JP. Nutrition care of patients with acute and chronic respiratory failure. Nutr Clin Pract. 1994;7:11–7.
This article considers the background as well as recommendations for the nutritional care of patients with acute and chronic respiratory failure.

Grote AE, Elwyn DH, Takala J, et al. Nutrition and metabolic effects of enteral and parenteral feeding on severely injured patients. Clin Nutr. 1987;6:161–7.

Jenkinson SG, Bryan CL. Solving the five main problems in nutrition for ventilated patients. J Crit Illness. 1991;6:243–50.

Mirtallo JM, Schneider PJ, Mavko K, et al. A comparison of essential and general amino acid infusions in the nutritional support of patients with compromised renal function. JPEN J Parenter Enteral Nutr. 1982;6:109–13.

In this study, use of essential amino acid solutions offered no advantage over general amino acid solutions.

Mullen JL, Buzby GP, Matthews DC, et al. Reduction of operative morbidity and mortality by combined preoperative and postoperative nutritional support. Ann Surg. 1980;139:160–7.

Schlichtig R, Sargent SC. Nutritional support of the mechanically ventilated patient. Crit Care Clin. 1990;6:767–84.

van den Berg B, Bogaard JM, Hop WC. High fat, low carbohydrate, enteral feeding in patients weaning from the ventilator. Intensive Care Med. 1994;20:470–5.

A study to see whether high-fat, low-carbohydrate enteral nutrition could reduce $\dot{V}_{CO_2}$ in patients during ventilator support and weaning from the ventilator in order to facilitate the weaning process.

Weinsier RL, Heimburger DC, Butterworth CE. Handbook of clinical nutrition. St. Louis: Mosby–Year Book; 1989.

An excellent manual for clinicians dealing with prevention, diagnosis, and management of nutritional problems.

Weinsier RL, Krumdieck CL. Death resulting from overzealous total parenteral nutrition: the refeeding syndrome revisited. Am J Clin Nutr. 1981;34:393–9.

Discusses how cachectic patients are relatively well adapted to their nutritionally deprived state. Aggressive refeeding results in hypophosphatemia and its associated disorders as well as in cardiac failure.

Wilmore DW. Alterations in protein, carbohydrate, and fat metabolism in injured and septic patients. J Am Coll Nutr. 1983;2:3–13.

Long-Term Mechanical Ventilation

O'Donohue WJ Jr, Giovannoni RM, Goldberg AI, et al. Long-term ventilation. Guidelines for management in the home and at alternate community sites. Report of Ad Hoc committee. Respiratory Care Section, American College of Chest Physicians. Chest. 1986;90:1–37S.

A review of medical assessment for long-term mechanical ventilation at home, factors important for patient selection, resources required, and hospital discharge criteria desirable before such initiation. A description of the delivery systems and monitoring devices, oxygen therapy, and nutritional support is outlined.

Financial Aspects and Prognosis of Patients on Mechanical Ventilation

Adams AB, Whitman J, Marcy T. Surveys of long-term ventilatory support in Minnesota: 1986 and 1992. Chest. 1993;103:1463–9.

Bernard GR, Artigas A, Brigham KL, et al. The American-European Consensus Conference on ARDS. Definitions, mechanisms, relevant outcomes, and clinical trial coordination. Am J Respir Crit Care Med. 1994;149:818–24.

Bowton DL, Goldsmith WM, Haponik EF. Substitution of metered-dose inhalers for hand-held nebulizers. Chest. 1992;101:305–8.

Byrick RJ, Minodorff C, McKee L, Mudge B. Cost-effectiveness of intensive care for respiratory failure patients. Crit Care Med. 1980;8:332–7.

Choi SC, Nelson LD. Kinetic therapy in critically ill patients: combined results based on meta-analysis. J Crit Care. 1992;7:57–62.

Civetta JM, Hudson-Civetta JA. Maintaining quality of care while reducing charges in the ICU: ten ways. Ann Surg. 1985;202:524-32.

Craven DE, Connolly MG Jr, Lichtenberg DA, et al. Contamination of mechanical ventilator with tubing changes every 24 or 48 hours. N Engl J Med. 1982;306:1505–9.

Davis H II, Lefrak SS, Miller D, Malt S. Prolonged mechanically assisted ventilation. An analysis of outcome and charges. JAMA. 1980;243:43–5.

Douglass PS, Rosen RL, Butler PW. DRG payment for long-term ventilator patients: implications and recommendations. Chest. 1987;91:415–7.

Dreyfuss D, Djedaini K, Weber P, et al. Prospective study of nosocomial pneumonia and of patient and circuit colonization during mechanical ventilation with circuit changes every 48 hours vs. no change. Am Rev Respir Dis. 1991;143:738–43.

Elpern EH, Silver MR, Rosen RL, et al. A cost effective approach for mechanically ventilated patients. Chest 1990;98(Suppl):75S.

Freichels T. Financial implications and recommendations for care of ventilator-dependent patients. J Nurs Admin. 1993;23:16–20.

Gay PC, Patel HG, Nelson SB, et al. Metered dose inhalers for bronchodilator delivery in intubated mechanically ventilated patients. Chest 1991;99:66–7.

Gracey DR, Gillespie D, Nobrega F, et al. Financial implication of prolonged ventilator care of Medicare patients under the prospective payment system: a multicenter study. Chest. 1987;91:424–7.

Knaus WA. Prognosis with mechanical ventilation: the influence of disease, severity of disease, age and chronic health status on survival from acute illness. Am Rev Respir Dis. 1989;140:S8–S13.

Kollef MH, Shapiro SD, Silver P, et al. A randomized, controlled trial of protocol-directed versus physician-directed weaning from mechanical ventilation. Crit Care Med. 1997;25:567–74.

Krieger BP. Economics of ventilator care. In: Tobin MJ, ed. Principles and practice of mechanical ventilation. New York: McGraw-Hill; 1994:1221–31.

Krieger BP, Ershowsky P, Spivak D, et al. Initial experience with a central respiratory monitoring unit as a cost-saving alternative to the intensive care unit for Medicare patients who require long-term ventilator support. Chest. 1988;93:395–7.

Latriano B, McCauley P, Astiz ME, et al. Non-ICU care of hemodynamically stable mechanically ventilated patients. Chest. 1996;1591–6.

Manzano JL, Lubillo S, Henriquez D, et al. Verbal communication of ventilator-dependent patients. Crit Care Med. 1993;212:512–7.

Menzies R, Gibbons W, Goldberg P. Determinants of weaning and survival among patients with COPD who require mechanical ventilation for acute respiratory failure. Chest. 1989;95:398–405.

Moss AH, Oppenheimer EA, Casey P, et al. Patients with amyotrophic lateral sclerosis receiving long-term mechanical ventilation: advance care planning and outcomes. Chest. 1996;110:249–55.

NIH Workshop Summary. Withholding and withdrawing mechanical ventilation. Am Rev Respir Dis. 1986;134:1327–30.

NIH Workshop Summary. Withholding and withdrawing mechanical ventilation. Am Rev Respir Dis. 1989;140:S1–S46.

Noseworthy T, Konopad E, Johnston R, et al. The cost of intensive care. Chest 1992;102(S):150S.

O'Donohue WJ, Giovannoni RM, Goldberg AI, et al. Long-term mechanical ventilation: guidelines for management in the home and at alternate community sites. Report of the Ad Hoc Committee, Respiratory Care Section, American College of Physicians. Chest. 1986;90(1)(Suppl):1S–37S.

Papadakis MA, Lee KK, Browner WS, et al. Prognosis of mechanically ventilated patients. West J Med. 1993;159:659–64.

Peters SG, Meadows JA, Gracey DR. Outcome of respiratory failure in hematologic malignancy. Chest. 1988;94:99–102.

Raoof S, Calves P, Mishra P, et al. One-year experience with the ventilator ward: financial and quality of care issues. Am Rev Respir Dis. 1991;143(Suppl):A684.

Rieves RD, Bass D, Carter RR, et al. Severe COPD and acute respiratory failure: correlates for survival at the time of tracheal intubation. Chest. 1993;104:854–60.

Rosen RL, Bone RC. Financial implications of ventilator care. Crit Care Clin. 1990;6:797–805.

Scheinhorn DJ, Artinian BM, Catlin JL. Weaning from prolonged mechanical ventilation: the experience at a regional weaning center. Chest. 1994;105:534–9.

Spivack D. The high cost of acute health care: a review of escalating costs and limitations of such exposure in intensive care units. Am Rev Respir Dis. 1987;136:1007–11.

Stauffer JL, Fayter NA, Graves B, et al. Survival following mechanical ventilation for acute respiratory failure in adult men. Chest. 1993;104:1222–9.

Swinburne AJ, Fedullo AJ, Shayne DS. Mechanical ventilation: analysis of increasing use and patient survival. J Intens Care Med. 1988;3:315–20.

Tablan OC, Anderson LJ, Arden NH, et al. Guidelines for prevention of nosocomial pneumonia. The Hospital Infection Control Practices Advisory Committee, Centers for Disease Control and Prevention. Infect Control Hosp Epidemiol. 1994;15:587–627.

Wachter RM, Luce JM, Safrin S, et al. Cost and outcome of intensive care for patients with AIDS, *Pneumocystis carinii* pneumonia, and severe respiratory failure. JAMA. 1995;273:230–5.

Wagner DP. Economics of prolonged mechanical ventilation. Am Rev Respir Dis. 1989;140:514–8.

Wandtke JC. Bedside chest radiography [Abstract] Radiology. 1994;190:1–10.

Index

A

A-a(O₂); *see* Alveolar-arterial oxygen gradient
ABGs; *see* Arterial blood gases
A/C mode; *see* Assist/control mode ventilation
Acidosis, respiratory, in cerebrovascular accident, 108
Acquired immune deficiency syndrome (AIDS), with *Pneumocystis* pneumonia, outcome-based studies in, 123
Acute respiratory distress, pressure volume curves in, 59
Acute respiratory failure
    comparative risk of dying from, 123
    noninvasive positive-pressure ventilation in, 37–40
Adult respiratory distress syndrome (ARDS)
    case study, 153–155
    outcome-based studies in, 123
    oxygenation in, management steps, 14
    prone positioning effects in, 44
    shear stress in, 94
    ventilation guidelines, 131–132
    ventilation problems, 107–108
    ventilation therapy quiz, 162
    volutrauma in, 92–93
Advance directives, 122–123
Age, survival and, 126
AIDS; *see* Acquired immune deficiency syndrome
Air, inspired, overheating of, 90
Airdyne air compressors, 90
Airway disease, ventilation guidelines in, 131
Airway management, 49–55
    airway cuff management, 54–55
    compliance and, 143
    intubation, 49–50
    medications, 50–51
        neuromuscular blocking agents, 52–54
    tracheostomy, 54
Airway obstruction, central, 131
Airway occlusion pressure, 72
Airway pressure release ventilation (APRV), 9, 29–30
Airways resistance, calculation, 60
Alarm failure, 89
Alarms sounding, troubleshooting, 110
Albumin, 114
Alkalosis
    metabolic, in acute asthma, 107
    respiratory, in cerebrovascular accident, 108
Alveolar gas equation, 147
Alveolar ventilation, formula, 147–148
Alveolar-arterial oxygen gradient [(A–a)O₂], 77
    formula, 147
Alveoli, shear stress and, 94
Analgesics, in airway management, 50–51
Annotated bibliography, 167–178
Apneic oxygenation, 45
APRV; *see* Airway pressure release ventilation
ARDS; *see* Adult respiratory distress syndrome
Arterial blood gases (ABGs)
    cost containment and, 121–122
    initial management, 134
    in permissive hypercapnia, 43
Arterial to alveolar O₂ tension (PaO₂/PAO₂), 77
Arterial to inspired O₂ ratio (PaO₂/FIO₂), 77
Arterial/alveolar oxygen tension ratio, formula, 148
Aseptic technique, in nosocomial pneumonia, 97
Aspiration, in acute asthma, 106

Assessment of need for ventilation, guidelines for, 131
Assist/control (A/C) mode ventilation, 9, 21, 22
    cardiovascular system effects of, 100
Asthma
    acute, ventilation problems in, 104–106
    auto-PEEP in, 62
    status asthmaticus case study, 150–151
    ventilation guidelines in, 132–133
Atelectasis, in acute asthma, 105, 106
Ativan (lorazepam), in airway management, 51
Augmented minute volume (mandatory minute ventilation), 27–28
Auto-PEEP
    in acute asthma, 104, 105
    in adult respiratory distress syndrome, 107
    avoiding development of, when increasing inspiratory time, 14
    causes, 62
    concept and definitions, 61
    diagrams, 139–140
    effects, 64–66
    measurement method, 63–64
    minimization strategies, 66–67
    practical example, 62
    practical tips, 67
    values of intrinsic PEEP clinically encountered, 62

B

Bacterial infections, in nosocomial pneumonia, 97
Barotrauma, 60, 91–92
Bear I and II adult volume ventilators, servicing, 90
Benzodiazepines, in acute asthma, 105
Bibliography, annotated, 167–178
Bilevel pressure ventilators (BiPAP), 9
    in noninvasive positive-pressure ventilation, 40
BiPAP; *see* Bilevel pressure ventilators
Bird oxygen blenders, 90
Bleeding, gastrointestinal, 103
Bleomycin, 103
Blood gases, arterial
    cost containment and, 121–122
    initial management, 134
    in permissive hypercapnia, 43
Boehringer respirometers, 90
Bourns Bear I and II adult volume ventilators, servicing, 90
Breathing
    paradoxic, 70
    rapid shallow, index of, 70
    spontaneous, trial of, in weaning, 80, 83
Bronchodilator therapy, efficacy of, 139
Bronchopleural fistula
    in adult respiratory distress syndrome, 108
    ventilation guidelines in, 133–134
Bronchospasm, in acute asthma, 105, 106
Burns, nutritional requirements in, 117

C

Calories, 113
    in nutritional therapy, 115, 116, 117, 118

Cancer
    nutritional requirements in, 117
    outcome-based studies in, 123
Carbohydrates, in nutritional therapy, 115–116
Carbon dioxide
    extracorporeal removal of, 45
    partial pressure, in arterial blood ($PaCO_2$)
        in acute asthma, 107
        in permissive hypercapnia, 43
        regulation, 4
    production ($\dot{V}CO_2$), 75
Cardiac arrest, outcome-based studies in, 123
Cardiac disorders, quiz on, 161
Cardiovascular system, ventilator mode effects on, 100
Case studies, 150–156
Central airway obstruction, 131
Central nervous system, weaning and, 69, 79
Cerebrovascular accident, ventilation problems in, 108
Chest x-rays, 122, 123
Chronic obstructive pulmonary disease (COPD)
    acute exacerbations, algorithm for ventilatory management of, 38
    auto-PEEP in, 62
    case study, 151–153
    outcomes in, 123, 127
    quiz on, 162–163
    ventilation guidelines in, 132–133
    ventilation problems in, 107
Circulatory failure, 131
CMV; see Controlled mode ventilation
Coma, 131
Communication, in home care, 129
Compliance, 58–59
    alarms sounding and, 110
    clinical settings, 143
    formulae, 148–149
    measurements
        applications, 59–61, 143
        exercise, 157
    quiz on, 160
    resistance and elasticity, 142
    weaning and, 73
Complications, 89–103; see also Problems with mechanical ventilation
    adverse effects of excessive pressure and flow rates, 91–96
    gastrointestinal, 103
    hemodynamic effects associated with mechanical ventilation, 99–100
    limitations of conventional ventilation, 89
    nosocomial pneumonia, 97–99
    nutritional, 103
    oxygen toxicity, 100–103
    prevention, cost containment and, 122
    psychological trauma, 103
    renal, 103
    side effects of adjuvant drugs, 103
    tracheal intubation, 103
    ventilator malfunction, 89–90
Concepts of mechanical ventilation, quiz on, 158
Consciousness, impaired, in nosocomial pneumonia, 99
Continuous positive airway pressure (CPAP)
    cardiovascular system effects of, 100
    positive end-expiratory pressure and, 35
    in site-specific ventilators, 9
Controlled mode ventilation (CMV), 21, 22
COPD; see Chronic obstructive pulmonary disease
Costs
    analysis of, 120
    of care for mechanically ventilated patients, 119–120
    containment, methods, 120–129
    reimbursement, 120, 128
CPAP; see Continuous positive airway pressure
CROP index, 78
Cuff leaks, in adult respiratory distress syndrome, 108
Cuff:trachea ratio, 54–55

D

Dead space volume to tidal volume ratio (VD/VT), 74
    formula, 149
Death, causes of, 127
Decreased-frequency ventilation, 41
Dehydration, in acute asthma, 104
Demographics, patient, survival and, 126
Diagnosis related groups (DRGs), 120
Diagrammatic representation, 135–146
Dialysis, nutritional requirements in, 117
Diaphragmatic electromyogram, 72
Dilaudid (hydromorphone), in airway management, 50–51
Diprivan (propofol), in airway management, 51
DRGs; see Diagnosis related groups
Drugs
    for airway management, 50–54
    side effects, 103
Duration of mechanical ventilation, minimizing, 120–121
Dynamic compliance, 58, 59, 148
Dynamic hyperinflation, definition, 61
Dysynchrony, patient-ventilator
    in acute asthma, 105, 106
    troubleshooting algorithm, 109

E

ECMO; see Extracorporeal membrane oxygenation
Economics, 119–129
Edema, pulmonary, auto-PEEP in, 62
Effective dynamic compliance, 58
Elasticity, 142
Electrolytes, weaning and, 69–70
Electromyogram, diaphragmatic, 72
Embolism, pulmonary, in acute asthma, 106
End-exhalation occlusion technique, 63
End-exhalation, increase of lung volume during, 5
End-expiration, increase of lung volume during, 5
End-inspiratory static pressures, 57–58
Endotracheal intubation, 49
Enteral nutrition, in nosocomial pneumonia, 98
Equations, 147–149
Ethics, of terminal withdrawal of ventilation, 86
Expenses; see Costs
Extended mandatory minute ventilation, 27–28
Extracorporeal CO_2 removal, 45
Extracorporeal membrane oxygenation (ECMO), 45
    venovenous access for, 48
Extubation, 83–84, 84

F

Fat, in nutritional assessment, 114
Fentanyl, in airway management, 50
Fick equation, 149
Financial aspects, 119–129
    cost analysis, 120
    cost of care, 119–120
    methods for curtailing costs, 120–129
    reimbursement, 120, 128
FIO_2; see Fractional concentration of oxygen in inspired gas
Flow rates
    excessive, adverse effects of, 91–96
    initial management, 134
    inspiratory time and, 144
Flow-by, 20
Flumazenil, in acute asthma, 105
Formulae, 147–149
Fractional concentration of oxygen in inspired gas (FIO_2)
    initial management, 134
    safe concentration, 101
    in site-specific ventilators, 9
Full face mask, in noninvasive positive-pressure ventilation, 38, 39

G

Gases
  alveolar gas equation, 147
  arterial blood
    cost containment and, 121–122
    initial management, 134
    in permissive hypercapnia, 43
  exchange of
    regulation, 4
    weaning and, 77–78
Gastric colonization, in nosocomial pneumonia, 99
Gastrointestinal complications, 103
Gender, survival and, 126
Glossary, 164–166
Glucose, 116
Guidelines in specific conditions, 131–134

H

Handwashing, in nosocomial pneumonia, 97
Head trauma, ventilation guidelines in, 133
Hemodynamics, 99–100
Hemoglobin, in oxygen toxicity, 100–101
Hemorrhage, gastrointestinal, 103
Hepatic encephalopathy, nutritional requirements in, 117
HFV; see High-frequency ventilation
High-frequency ventilation (HFV), 32–33, 41
Home care, 128–129
Home care ventilators, 8, 9
Hospital resources, rationing, 122–123
Host defenses, in malnutrition, 112
Humidification, inadequate, 89
Humidification system, in site-specific ventilators, 9
Hydromorphone, in airway management, 50–51
Hypercapnia
  in acute asthma, 106
  permissive, 42–43
Hypercapnic respiratory failure, 66
Hyperinflation, dynamic, definition, 61
Hyperoxia, 100–103
Hyperventilation
  in acute asthma, 107
  in cerebrovascular accident, 108
Hypotension
  in acute asthma, 104–105, 106
  in adult respiratory distress syndrome, 107
Hypoventilation, in cerebrovascular accident, 108
Hypoxemia
  in acute asthma, 106
  in acute respiratory distress syndrome, 107
  initial ventilator set-up in, 16
  reversal of, 4
  troubleshooting, 110–111
Hypoxemic respiratory failure, noninvasive positive-pressure
    ventilation in, 37

I

ICU costs, 119; see also Financial aspects
ICU ventilators, 8, 9
  in noninvasive positive-pressure ventilation, 39
Immobility, in nosocomial pneumonia, 98
Indications, 3
Infections, in nosocomial pneumonia, 97
Initial ventilator set-up, 15–20
Initial ventilatory support, 134
  quiz on, 159
Inspiration:expiration ratio, initial management, 134
Inspiratory flow
  inappropriate, 138
  in initial ventilator set-up
    effects, 16–18

profile, 18–19
rate, 16
Inspiratory pressure, peak; see Peak inspiratory pressure
Inspiratory time
  effects of inspiratory flows on, 16
  flow rates and, 144
  formula, 149
  increasing, 14
Integrative indices, weaning and, 78
Intensive care unit costs, 119; see also Financial aspects
Intensive care unit ventilators, 8, 9
  in noninvasive positive-pressure ventilation, 39
Intravascular oxygenation, 45, 47
Intrinsic PEEP; see Auto-PEEP
Intubation, 49–50
  in nosocomial pneumonia, 98
  right main stem, in acute asthma, 104, 105, 106
  tracheal, complications, 103
  translaryngeal, tracheostomy vs., 54
Inverse ratio ventilation, 25–26
  cardiovascular system effects of, 100
IRV; see Inverse ratio ventilation
Ischemia, myocardial, ventilation guidelines in, 133

J

Juxtacardiac pressure, 68

K

Kwashiorkor, 113, 114, 117

L

Laplace law, 65
Left ventricular failure, case study, 155–156
Legal aspects, of terminal withdrawal of ventilation, 86, 87
LFPPV-ECCO$_2$R; see Low-frequency positive-pressure ventilation
    and extracorporeal CO$_2$ removal
Lipids, in nutritional therapy, 115–116, 117
Liquid ventilation, 46, 47
Liver disease, nutritional requirements in, 117
Lorazepam, in airway management, 51
Low-frequency positive-pressure ventilation and extracorporeal
    CO$_2$ removal (LFPPV-ECCO$_2$R), 45
Lung parenchyma, 56, 57, 131
  compliance and, 143
Lung volumes, increasing, 5
Lungs
  mechanics, 56–61
  overdistension, 93, 137
  weaning and, 79

M

Machine failure, 89
Malnutrition; see also Nutrition
  clinical significance of, 112
  protein, 113, 117
  role of nutritional repletion in, 113
Mandatory minute ventilation (MMV), 27–28
Marasmus, 113, 117
Masks, in noninvasive positive-pressure ventilation, 38–39
Maximum inspiratory pressure, 70
Maximum voluntary ventilation (MVV), 74
Mechanical ventilation
  case studies, 150–156
  example of patient on, 144
  guidelines in specific conditions, 131–134
  indications, 3

Mechanical ventilation—cont'd
    modes; *see* Modes of ventilation
      objectives, 4–5
      quiz on, 158–163
      reasons for increased use of, 119
Medicaid reimbursement, 128
Medicare reimbursement, 120, 128
Medications
    for airway management, 50–54
    side effects, 103
Metabolic alkalosis, in acute asthma, 107
Metabolism, nutritional therapy and, 116
Meteorism, 103
Metered dose inhalers, cost containment and, 122
Midazolam, in airway management, 51
Minute ventilation ($\dot{V}E$), 73, 134
MMV; *see* Mandatory minute ventilation
Modes of ventilation, 21–33, 41
    airway pressure release, 29–30
    assist/control, 21, 22
    cardiovascular system effects of, 100
    controlled, 21, 22
    high-frequency, 32–33
    inverse ratio, 25–26
    mandatory minute, 27–28
    in noninvasive positive-pressure ventilation, 39
    pressure support, 23–24
    pressure-targeted vs. volume-targeted, 11–13
    proportional assist, 31
    quiz on, 159–160
    for site-specific ventilators, 9
    synchronous intermittent mandatory, 21, 22
Monitoring, 56–68
    auto-PEEP
      causes, 62
      concept and definitions, 61
      effects, 64–66
      measurement method, 63–64
      minimization strategies, 66–67
      practical example, 62
      practical tips, 67
      values of intrinsic PEEP clinically encountered, 62
    after extubation, 84
    influence of PEEP on pulmonary artery occlusion pressure or
      wedge pressure, 67–68
    lung mechanics
      compliance, 58–59
      compliance measurements applications, 59–61
      conducting unit, 56
      lung parenchyma, 56
      peak inspiratory pressures, 56–57
      plateau pressures or end-inspiratory static pressures, 57–58
Morphine
    in acute asthma, 105
    in airway management, 50
Mortality, causes of, 127
Muscle mass, in nutritional assessment, 114
Muscle strength, respiratory, weaning and, 70–72, 79, 134
MVV; *see* Maximum voluntary ventilation
Myocardial ischemia, ventilation guidelines in, 133
Myocardial oxygen consumption, lowering, 5

N

Naloxone, in acute asthma, 105
Narcotics, in acute asthma, 105
Nasal mask, in noninvasive positive-pressure ventilation, 38, 39
Nasotracheal intubation, 49
Nebulization, inadequate, 89
Negative-pressure ventilators, 8
Neuromuscular blocking agents, in airway management, 52–54
Neuromuscular disease
    assessment of need for ventilation in, 131

quiz on, 161
ventilation guidelines in, 133
NIPPV; *see* Noninvasive positive-pressure ventilation
Nitric oxide inhalation, 46
Nitrogen balance, 114–115, 118
    formula, 149
Noninvasive positive-pressure ventilation (NIPPV)
    in acute respiratory failure, 37–40
    in weaning, 81
Norcuron (vecuronium), in airway management, 52
Nosocomial pneumonia, 97–99
Nurses, responsibilities of, 126
Nursing home residents, survival of, 127
Nutrition, 112–118
    assessment, 114–115
    clinical significance of malnutrition, 112
    complications, 103
    disorders, 113–114
    nature of problem, 112
    in nosocomial pneumonia, 98
    requirements, 117
      increased, causes of, 112
    role of repletion in malnourished states, 113
    support in protein malnutrition, 117
    therapy
      prescription selection, 116–118
      principles, 115–116
    weaning and, 70

O

O_2; *see* Oxygen
Objectives, 4–5
Obstructive airways disease; *see also* Asthma; Chronic obstructive
      pulmonary disease
    ventilation guidelines in, 132–133
Occult PEEP; *see* Auto-PEEP
Orotracheal intubation, 49
Outcomes, 123–124, 126–127
Overdistention, 93, 137
Overfeeding, 112, 115, 116, 117
Overheating of inspired air, 90
Oxygen
    concentration, in initial ventilator set-up, 16
    fractional concentration in inspired gas (FIO_2)
      initial management, 134
      safe concentration, 101
      in site-specific ventilators, 9
    partial pressure, in arterial blood (PaO_2)
      in adult respiratory distress syndrome, prone positioning
        and, 44
      ratio to fractional concentration of oxygen in inspired gas,
        77
      ratio to partial pressure of oxygen in alveolar gas, 77
      regulation, 4
    supply, in home care, 129
    toxicity, 100–103
    weaning indices, 76–77
Oxygen consumption
    formula, 149
    myocardial, lowering, 5
Oxygen content, formula, 149
Oxygen cost of breathing, 76–77
Oxygen saturation, arterial blood (SaO_2), regulation, 4
Oxygen tension ratio, arterial/alveolar, formula, 148
Oxygenation
    in adult respiratory distress syndrome, management steps, 14
    extracorporeal membrane, 45, 48
    factors affecting, 13
    failure, 1
    new techniques in, 45–48
    weaning and, 134

P

PaCO$_2$; *see* Partial pressure of carbon dioxide in arterial blood
Pancuronium, in airway management, 52, 53
PaO$_2$; *see* Partial pressure of oxygen in arterial blood
PaO$_2$/FIO$_2$; *see* Arterial to inspired O$_2$ ratio
PAOP; *see* Pulmonary artery occlusion pressure
PaO$_2$/PAO$_2$; *see* Arterial to alveolar O$_2$ tension
Paradoxic breathing, 70
Partial liquid ventilation, 46, 47
Partial pressure of carbon dioxide, in arterial blood (PaCO$_2$)
    in acute asthma, 107
    in permissive hypercapnia, 43
    regulation, 4
Partial pressure of oxygen in arterial blood (PaO$_2$)
    in adult respiratory distress syndrome, prone positioning and, 44
    ratio to fractional concentration of oxygen in inspired gas, 77
    ratio to partial pressure of oxygen in alveolar gas, 77
    regulation, 4
Patient demographics, survival and, 126
Patient-ventilator dyssynchrony
    in acute asthma, 105, 106
    troubleshooting algorithm, 109
Patient-ventilator interface
    in home care, 129
    in noninvasive positive-pressure ventilation, 38, 40
PAV; *see* Proportional assist ventilation
Pavulon (pancuronium), in airway management, 52, 53
Peak airway pressure and flow, waveform pattern, 141
Peak inspiratory pressure (PIP), 56–57, 58
    in acute asthma, 105–106
    in adult respiratory distress syndrome, 107
    airways resistance and, 60
    barotrauma and, 60, 91
    in effective dynamic compliance, 59
    effects of inspiratory flows on, 17
PEEP; *see* Positive end-expiratory pressure
Pel; *see* Plateau pressure
Perflubron, 46
Permissive hypercapnia, 42–43
Personnel, 126
Physicians, responsibilities of, 126
PImax; *see* Maximum inspiratory pressure
PIP; *see* Peak inspiratory pressures
Plateau pressure (Pel), 57–58
    in adult respiratory distress syndrome, 107
    airways resistance and, 60
    auto-PEEP and, 64
    barotrauma and, 60
    in static compliance, 59
Pleural pressure, mean, in estimation of juxtacardiac pressure, 68
Pneumonia
    in acute asthma, 106
    nosocomial, 97–99
Pneumothorax, in acute asthma, 104, 105, 106
Portable pressure ventilators, in noninvasive positive-pressure ventilation, 40
Positive end-expiratory pressure (PEEP), 34
    alveoli and, 145
    auto–; *see* Auto-PEEP
    cardiovascular system effects of, 100
    continuous positive airway pressure and, 35
    diagrams, 145–146
    effects, 146
    influence on pulmonary artery occlusion pressure or wedge pressure on, 67–68
    in minimizing auto-PEEP, 66–67
    optimal, calculating, 60
    passive inflation pressures recorded with supersyringe technique, 36, 95–96
    quiz on, 159–160
    in site-specific ventilators, 9
Positive-pressure ventilation
    in home care, 129
    noninvasive
        in acute respiratory failure, 37–40
        in weaning, 81
Positive-pressure ventilators, 7, 8
Postoperative ventilation guidelines, 133
Pressure; *see also specific types*
    excessive, adverse effects of, 91–96
Pressure assist/control, 9
Pressure control waveform, 136
Pressure MMV, 9
Pressure SIMV, 9
Pressure support, calculating, 61
Pressure volume curves
    in acute respiratory distress etiology, 59
    loop, 139
    in lung overdistention, 137
    in shear stress, 95–96
Pressure-support ventilation (PSV), 9, 23–24
    in weaning, 80, 83
Pressure-targeted ventilation
    in home care, 129
    volume-targeted ventilation vs., 11–13
Problems with mechanical ventilation, 104–108; *see also* Complications
    in acute asthma, 104–106
    in adult respiratory distress syndrome, 107–108
    in cerebrovascular accident, 108
    in chronic obstructive pulmonary disease, 107
    troubleshooting, 109–111
Prognosis, 123–124, 126–127
Prone position ventilation, 43–44
Propofol, in airway management, 51
Proportional assist ventilation (PAV), 31
Protective equipment, in nosocomial pneumonia, 97
Protein(s)
    malnutrition, 113, 117
    in nutritional therapy, 116, 117, 118
    requirements, 117
    visceral, 113, 114
PSV; *see* Pressure-support ventilation
Psychological trauma, 103
Pulmonary artery occlusion pressure (PAOP), influence of positive end-expiratory pressure on, 67–68
Pulmonary capillaries, weaning and, 79
Pulmonary edema, auto-PEEP in, 62
Pulmonary embolism, in acute asthma, 106
Puritan Bennett MA-1 adult volume ventilators, servicing, 90
Puritan Bennett 7200A/AE microprocessor ventilators, servicing, 90

Q

Q̇s/Q̇T; *see* Shunt fraction
Quiz, 158–163

R

Radiology, chest x-rays, 122, 123
Rapid shallow breathing, index of, 70
Rationing hospital resources, 122–123
REE; *see* Resting energy expenditure
Reimbursement, 120, 128
Renal complications, 103
Renal failure, nutritional requirements in, 117
Resistance, 142
    formula, 147
Respiratory acidosis, in cerebrovascular accident, 108
Respiratory alkalosis, in cerebrovascular accident, 108
Respiratory alternans, 71
Respiratory care units, step-down, 124
Respiratory failure
    assessment of need for ventilation in, 131
    classification, 1
    comparative risk of dying from, 123

Respiratory failure—cont'd
  components of respiratory system and, 2
  hypercapnic, 66
  noninvasive positive-pressure ventilation in, 37–40
  nutritional requirements in, 117
  severe, clinical signs of, 3
Respiratory gas exchange, weaning and, 77–78
Respiratory muscle demands, weaning and, 73–77, 79
Respiratory muscle strength, weaning and, 70–72, 79, 134
Respiratory rate (RR), 74
  in initial ventilator set-up, 15
Respiratory system, in malnutrition, 112
Respiratory therapists, responsibilities of, 126
Resting energy expenditure (REE), 114
Retinol-binding protein, 114
RR; see Respiratory rate
RR/VT; see Rapid shallow breathing, index of

S

SaO$_2$; see Oxygen saturation, arterial blood
Secretions, in acute asthma, 105
Sedatives
  in acute asthma, 105
  in airway management, 51
Sepsis, nutritional requirements in, 117
Shear stress, 94–95
Shunt fraction (Q̇s/Q̇T), 78
  formula, 148
Simplified weaning index, 78
SIMV; see Synchronized intermittent mandatory ventilation
Sisatracurium, in airway management, 53
Site-specific ventilators, 8–9
Spontaneous breathing trial, in weaning, 80, 83
Spontaneous ventilation, cardiovascular system effects of, 100
Staffing, 126
Static compliance, 58, 73, 149
Status asthmaticus, case study, 150–151
Step-down units, 124
Stroke, ventilation problems in, 108
Stupor, 131
Sublimaze (fentanyl), in airway management, 50
Supersyringe technique, 36, 95
Survival, 123, 126–127
Synchronized intermittent mandatory ventilation (SIMV), 21, 22
  cardiovascular system effects of, 100
  waveform patterns, 135–136
  in weaning, 80, 83

T

Techniques of ventilation and oxygenation, newer, 41–48
Terminal withdrawal, 86–88
  quiz on, 161–162
Thyroxin-binding prealbumin, 114
Tidal volume (VT)
  in initial ventilator set-up, 15
  in permissive hypercapnia, 42, 43
  during pressure-targeted ventilation, factors affecting, 13
Toxicity, oxygen, 100–103
Tracheal insufflation of oxygen (TRIO), 45
Tracheal intubation, complications, 103
Tracheomalacia, in adult respiratory distress syndrome, 108
Tracheostomy, 54
Tracheostomy tubes
  in home care, 129
  trials, in weaning, 80–81, 83
Transferrin, 114
Transfers to long-term facilities, 125
Translaryngeal intubation, tracheostomy vs., 54
Transport ventilators, 8, 9
Trauma
  barotrauma, 60, 91–92

head, ventilation guidelines in, 133
  nutritional requirements in, 117
  psychological, 103
  volutrauma, 92–93
Trigger sensitivity, in initial ventilator set-up, 20
TRIO; see Tracheal insufflation of oxygen
Troubleshooting, 109–111
T-tubes
  in home care, 129
  trials, in weaning, 80–81, 83

U

Underfeeding, 117

V

Vascular access, for extracorporeal membrane oxygenation, 48
VC; see Vital capacity
V̇CO$_2$; see Volume of carbon dioxide production per minute
VD/VT; see Dead space volume to tidal volume ratio
V̇E; see Minute ventilation
Vecuronium, in airway management, 52, 53
Vegetative state, persistent, terminal withdrawal of ventilation in, 86–88
Venovenous access, for extracorporeal membrane oxygenation, 48
Ventilation modes; see Modes of ventilation
Ventilator circuit, cost containment and, 122
Ventilator set-up, initial, 15–20
  inspiratory flow
    effects, 16–18
    profile, 18–19
    rate, 16
  oxygen concentration, 16
  respiratory rate, 15
  settings, 134
  tidal volume, 15
  trigger sensitivity, 20
Ventilators
  initial management, 134
    quiz on, 159
  malfunction and preventive maintenance, 89–90
  types of, 7–9
    in noninvasive positive-pressure ventilation, 39, 40
    quiz on, 158–159
Ventilatory demands and mechanics, weaning and, 134
Ventilatory failure, 1
Ventilatory support; see Mechanical ventilation
Versed (midazolam), in airway management, 51
Vital capacity (VC), 71
Volume assist/control, 9
Volume MMV, 9
Volume of carbon dioxide production per minute (V̇CO$_2$), 75
Volume SIMV, 9
Volume-targeted ventilation, 65
  in home care, 129
  pressure-targeted ventilation vs., 11–13
Volutrauma, 92–93
VT; see Tidal volume

W

Waveforms
  decelerating
    with inspiratory hold time, 138
    normal, 140
    typical control, indicating flow and volume, 140
  peak airway pressure and flow, 141
  pressure control, 136
  SIMV ventilation patterns, 135–136
    inspiratory, 19
    in pressure-targeted vs. volume-targeted ventilation, 12

Weaning, 69–85
  definition and criteria, 69
  extubation protocol guidelines, 83–84
  factors to correct before, 69–79
  guidelines, 69, 83
  indices, 60, 70–78, 79
  methods, 79–82
  parameters monitored after extubation, 83–84
  quiz on, 160
  to shorten duration of mechanical ventilation, 121

  successful, criteria suggesting, 134
  terminal, 86–88
    quiz on, 161–162
  unsuccessful, algorithm, 85
Wedge pressure, influence of positive end-expiratory pressure on,
    67–68
WOB; *see* Work of breathing
Work of breathing (WOB), 75–76
Wright respirometers, 90

ABOUT THE AUTHORS

Suhail Raoof, MD, FACP, FCCP

Dr. Suhail Raoof, who graduated from Maulana Azad Medical College, Delhi University, India, is Assistant Professor of Medicine at the State University of New York at Stony Brook and has been Director of the Medical Intensive Care Unit at Nassau County Medical Center in East Meadow, New York, for more than five years. He has been involved in many clinical and basic research projects, some of which have been nominated for awards at a national level. He has more than 30 abstracts and 10 publications in peer-reviewed journals to his credit. He has been Co-director of the Mechanical Ventilation Workshop at the Annual Session of the American College of Physicians since 1991, and Director of the two-day Annual Mechanical Ventilation Workshop for three consecutive years.

Faroque A. Khan, MB, MACP, FCCP, FRCP(C)

Dr. Faroque A. Khan, a graduate of Medical College, Srinagar, Kashmir, is the Chairman of the Department of Medicine and Program Director of the Internal Medicine Program at Nassau County Medical Center, East Meadow, New York, and is Professor of Medicine at the State University of New York at Stony Brook. Dr. Khan was awarded Mastership in the American College of Physicians in 1993. He has written more than 100 articles and 130 abstracts and has also contributed chapters to various medical textbooks. In addition, Dr. Khan has been the principal investigator of several clinical studies, receiving 35 grants totaling more than 2 million dollars from the World Health Organization, National Institutes of Health, and other educational institutions. Dr. Khan has been Director of the Mechanical Ventilation Workshop at the Annual Session of the American College of Physicians since 1988.